A Manual of the
Operations of Surgery

A Manual of the Operations of Surgery
Copyright © 2000 BiblioBazaar
All rights reserved

The present edition is a reproduction of a previous publication of this work. Minor typographical errors may have been corrected without note; however, for with most typographic layout, spelling, punctuation and capitalization have been retained from the original text.

ISBN: 978-1-64799-145-6

Joseph Bell

A Manual of the Operations of Surgery

ISBN: 978-1-64799-145-6

CONTENTS

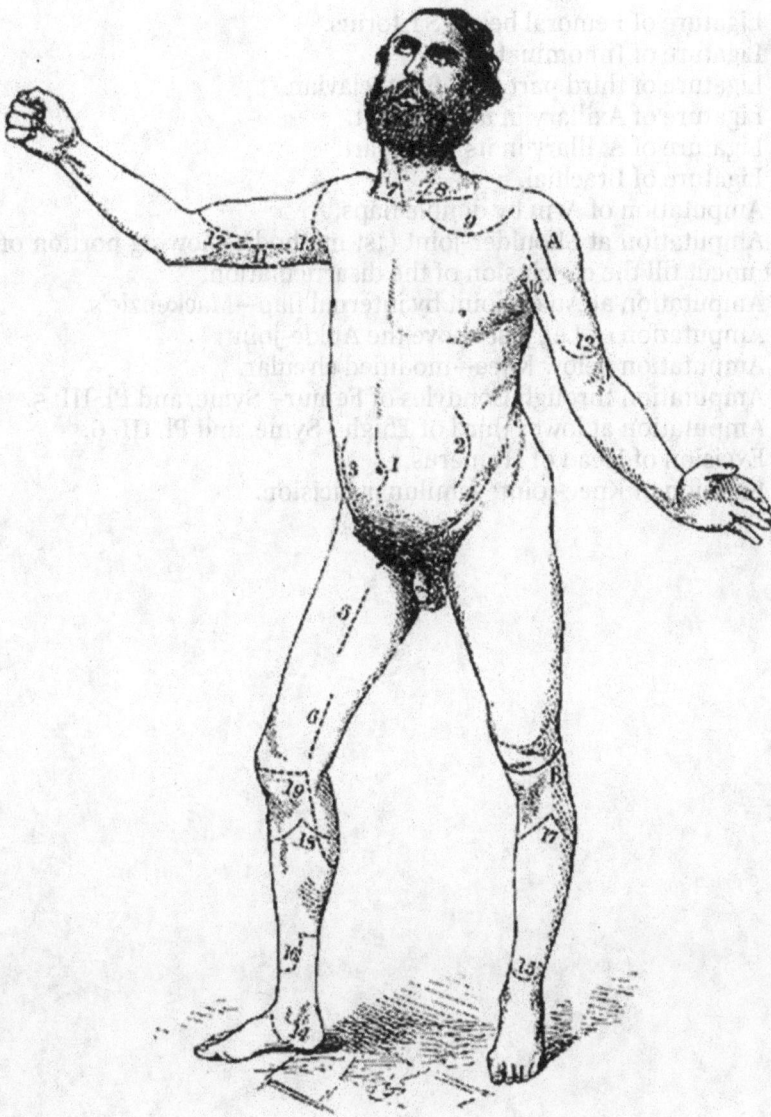

PLATE I

1. Ligature of Aorta—Sir A. Cooper's incision.
2. Ligature of Aorta—South and Murray's incision.
3. Ligature of Common Iliac.
4. Ligature of External Iliac—Sir A. Cooper's.
5. Ligature of Femoral in Scarpa's triangle.

---

[1] This line is placed too low down; it should be in the middle third of the thigh.

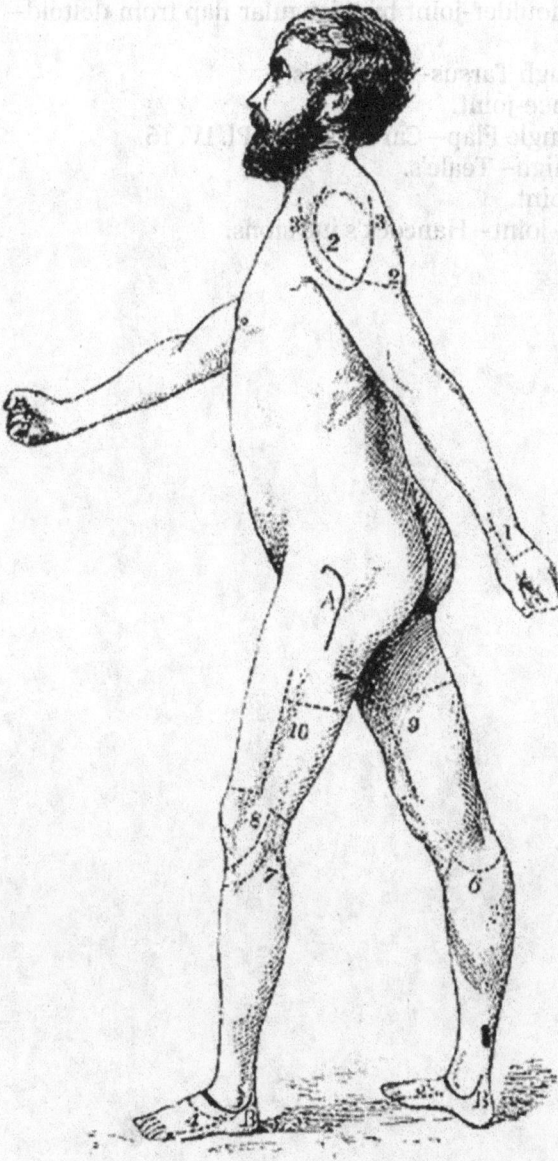

PLATE II

1.   Amputation at lower third of Fore-arm—Teale's.
2-2.   Amputation at Shoulder-joint by large postero-external flap—
2d method.

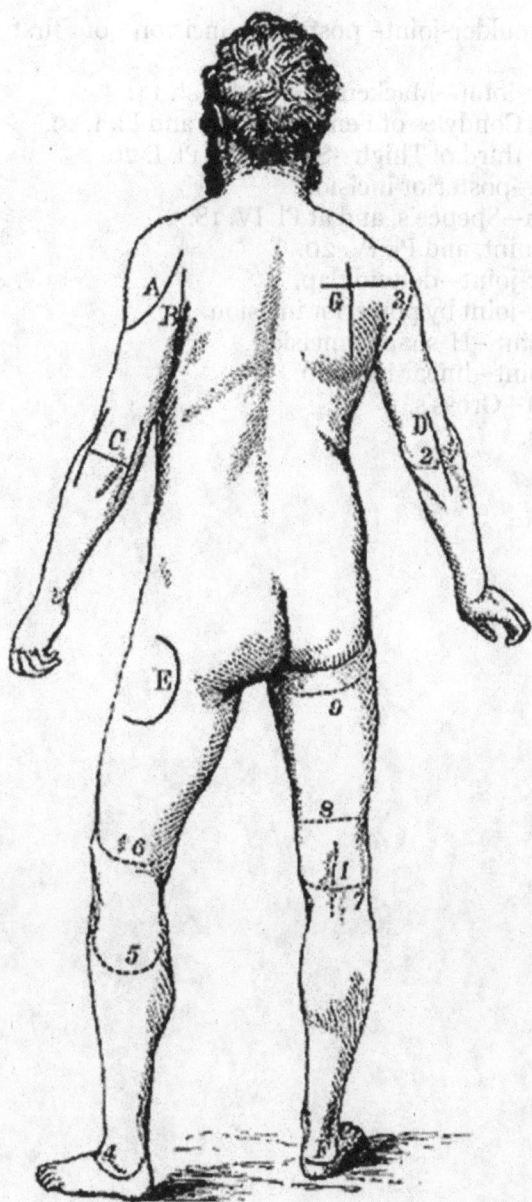

PLATE III

1.   Ligature of Popliteal.
2.   Amputation at Elbow-joint—posterior flap.

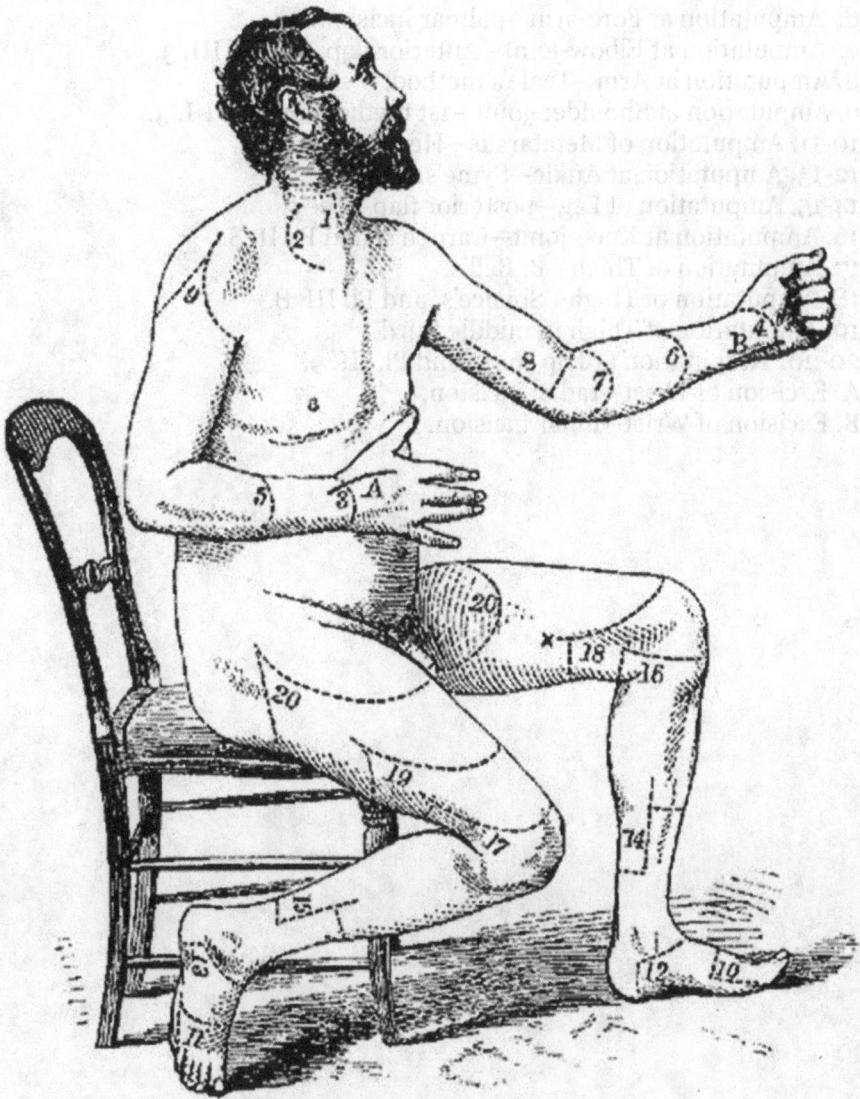

PLATE IV

1. Ligature of Carotid.
2. Ligature of Subclavian (3d stage)—Skey's incision.
3. Amputation at Wrist-joint—dorsal incision.
4. Amputation at Wrist-joint—palmar incision.
5. Amputation at Fore-arm—dorsal incision.

CHAPTER I

LIGATURE OF ARTERIES

Ligature of Arteries.—In a work of this nature there is no room for any discussion of the principles which should guide us in the selection of cases, or of the pathology of aneurism, or the local effects of the ligature on the vessels. One or two fundamental axioms may be given in a few words:—

1. In selecting the spot for the application of the ligature, avoid as far as possible bifurcations, or the neighbourhood of large collateral branches.

2. A free incision should be made through the skin and subjacent textures, till the sheath of the artery is reached and fairly exposed.

3. The sheath must be opened and the artery cleaned with a sharp knife till the white external coat is clearly seen. The portion cleaned should, however, be as small as possible, consistent with thorough exposure, so that the ligature may be passed round the vessel without force.

4. As the artery should never be raised from its bed, it is generally advisable to pass the needle only so far as just to permit the eye to be seen past the vessel. The ligature should then be seized by a pair of forceps and gently pulled through, the needle being cautiously withdrawn. When catgut is used, it is better to pass the unarmed needle till the eye is visible, then thread and withdraw it, thus pulling the catgut through.

5. As a rule, the needle should be passed from the side of the vessel at which the chief dangers exist. This will generally be in the side at which the vein is.

6. The ligature should be single, and consist of strong well-waxed silk, and should always be drawn as tight as possible, so as to divide the internal and middle coats of the vessel. In cases where the wound is to be treated with antiseptic precautions and an attempt at immediate union made, the ligature may be of strong catgut properly prepared, and both ends of it may be cut off.

7. Before the ligature is tightened, it is well to feel that pressure between the ligature and the finger arrests the pulsation of the tumour.

Ligature of the Aorta.—It has been found necessary in a few rare cases to place a ligature on the abdominal aorta; no case has as yet survived the operation beyond a very few days, but they have in their progress sufficiently proved that the circulation can be carried on, and gangrene does not necessarily result even after such a decided interference with vascular supply.

Operation.—The ligature may be applied in one of two ways, the choice being influenced by the nature of the disease for which it is done.

1. A straight incision (Plate I. fig. 1) in the linea alba, just avoiding the umbilicus by a curve, and dividing the peritoneum, allows the intestines to be pushed aside, and the aorta exposed still covered by the peritoneum, as it lies in front of the lumbar vertebræ. The peritoneum must again be divided very cautiously at the point selected, and the aortic plexus of nerves carefully dissected off, in order that they may not be interfered with by the ligature. The ligature should then be passed round, tied, cut short, and the wound accurately sewed up.

2. Without wounding the peritoneum.

A curved incision (Plate I. fig. 2), with its convexity backwards, from the projecting end of the tenth rib to a point a little in front of the anterior superior spinous process of the ilium. At first through the skin and fascia only, this incision must be continued through the muscles of the abdominal wall, one by one, till the transversalis fascia is exposed, which must then be scraped through very cautiously, so as not to injure the peritoneum, which is to be detached from the fascia covering the psoas and iliacus muscles, and must be held inwards and out of the way by bent copper spatulæ. The common iliac will then be felt pulsating, and on it the finger may easily be guided up until the aorta is reached.

The really difficult part of the operation now begins: to isolate the vessel from the spine behind, the inferior cava on the right side, and the plexus of nerves in the cellular tissue all round. The cleaning of the vessel must be done in great measure by the finger-nail, and much dexterity will be required to pass the ligature without unnecessarily raising the vessel from its bed, especially as the vessel itself may very possibly be diseased, and the aneurism of the iliac trunk for which the operation is required will displace and confuse the parts, and may have set up adhesive inflammation.

Results.—Operation has been performed at least ten times. By the first method by Sir Astley Cooper and Mr. James; by the second by Drs. Murray and Monteiro, M'Guire, Heron Watson, and Stokes, and Mr. South, and Czerny of Heidelberg. All the cases proved fatal; Dr. Monteiro's survived for ten days, and eventually perished from hæmorrhage; the rest all died at shorter intervals.

Ligature of Common Iliac.—Anatomical Note.—This short thick trunk varies slightly in its relations on the two sides of the body. As the aorta bifurcates on the left side of the body of the fourth lumbar vertebra, the common iliac of the right side would have a longer course to pursue than that on the left, if both ended at corresponding points. However, this is not always the case, as has been pointed out by Mr. Adams of Dublin, as the right common iliac often bifurcates sooner than the left does. With this slight difference, the position of the two vessels is precisely similar, each extending along the brim of the pelvis

2

from the bifurcation of the aorta towards the sacro-iliac synchondrosis for about two inches. Sometimes the division takes place a little higher, even at the junction of the last lumbar vertebra and the sacrum. This variation depends chiefly on the length of the artery, which, as Quain has shown, varies from one inch and a half to more than three inches.

The anterior surface of both arteries is covered by the peritoneum, and each is crossed by the ureter just as it bifurcates into its branches.

The artery of the right side is in close contact behind with its corresponding vein, which at its upper part projects to the outside, and below to the inner side. The artery of the left side is less involved with its vein, which lies below it, and to the inside. The right is in contact with a coil of ileum, the left with the colon. The inferior mesenteric artery crosses the left one, while to the outside of both, and behind them, lie the sympathetic and obdurator nerves.

There are no named branches from the common iliac.

Operation.—The chief difficulties to be encountered are—1. The close proximity of the peritoneum, and specially the risk there is that it has become adherent to the sac of the aneurism; 2. The depth of the parts, and tendency of the intestines to roll into the wound; 3. Specially on the right side, the proximity of the great veins. With these exceptions the passing of the ligature is not so difficult as in some situations, the lax cellular tissue in which the vessel lies generally yielding much more easily than the tough sheath which elsewhere, as in the femoral, requires accurate dissection.

Incision.—(Plate I. fig. 3.)—From a point about half an inch above the centre of Poupart's ligament, a crescentic incision should be made, at first extending upwards and outwards, so as to pass about one inch inside of the anterior superior spine of the ilium, and then prolonged upwards and inwards, as far as may be rendered necessary by the size of the aneurism or the depth of parts. It must extend through skin and superficial fascia, exposing the tendon of the external oblique, which must then be slit up to the full extent visible. The spermatic cord may then be easily exposed under the edge of the internal oblique, and the forefinger of the left hand inserted on the cord, and thus beneath the internal oblique and transversalis muscles, the peritoneum being quite safe below.

On the finger these muscles may be safely divided to the full extent of the external incision. The deep circumflex iliac artery if possible should not be divided, but may bleed smartly and require a ligature.

The peritoneum must then be very cautiously raised from the tumour, and supported, along with the intestines, by copper spatulæ. The surgeon will rarely succeed in obtaining anything like a satisfactory view of the vessel, but can expose it for the ligature by the aid of his

3

finger-nail. An ordinary aneurism-needle will generally suffice for the conveyance of the ligature.

The difficulties may occasionally be much increased by special circumstances, such as great stoutness of the patient, and consequent thickness of the abdominal wall; or large size of the aneurism, which may cause alterations in the relation of parts and adhesion of the peritoneum. The ureter generally gives no trouble, as in pressing back the peritoneum it is adherent to it, and is removed along with it towards the middle line.

Results.—Are not by any means satisfactory.

Out of twenty-two cases in which the common iliac has been tied for aneurism, eight recovered and fourteen died; while out of thirteen cases where it required ligature for hæmorrhage after amputation, rupture of aneurism, etc., only one recovered.

Ligature of Internal Iliac.—Little need be added to the account just given of the operation for ligature of the common iliac, as precisely the same incisions are required. The operator having reached the bifurcation of the vessel, must, instead of tracing it upwards, endeavour to trace it downwards, and the same time inwards, into the basin of the pelvis. To do this his finger must cross the external iliac artery, which will pulsate under the joint of the ungual phalanx, while the pulp of the finger is touching the internal iliac,—the external iliac vein, which occupies the angle formed by the bifurcation of the artery, lying between these two points. The ligature should be applied within three-quarters of an inch from the bifurcation.

Anatomical Note.—This short thick trunk extends backwards and inwards (Ellis); downwards and backwards (Harrison), in front of the sacro-iliac synchondrosis, as far as the upper extremity of the great sacro-sciatic notch, a distance varying in the adult from one and a half to two inches in length. It forms a curve with its concavity forwards, and at its termination divides into, rather than gives off, its two or three principal branches. Its corresponding vein is in close contact behind, as also the lumbo-sacral nerve, the obdurator nerve to its outer side. The peritoneum covers it anteriorly, and it is crossed just at its commencement by the ureter. On the left side it is covered anteriorly by the rectum. Of its anatomical relations, that of the external iliac vein is perhaps the most important, as it is apt to interfere with the passing of the needle.

Results.—This vessel has been tied for aneurism of one or other of its branches, or for wound, about seventeen times.[2] Of these seven recovered; in ten the operation proved fatal, in most of them from secondary hæmorrhage. In one case the hæmorrhage occurred within twelve hours after the operation. The circulation of the parts supplied after the ligature is carried on mainly by the lumbar and lateral sacral

---

[2] Erichsen, Surgery. Sixth edition, vol. ii. p. 121.

branches, which become much developed even before the operation, in cases of aneurism.

Ligature of External Iliac.—Anatomical Note.—This artery extends from the bifurcation of the common iliac to the centre of Poupart's ligament, where it leaves the abdomen, passing under the ligament, and becomes the common femoral. Its upper extremity is thus not always constant, varying in position from the sacro-lumbar fibro-cartilage to the upper end of the sacro-iliac synchondrosis, or even a little lower down. Thus, though the position of the lower end is at a fixed point, the artery varies in length. In an adult male of moderate stature it is from three and a half to four inches in length. On the surface of the abdomen the position of this vessel would be indicated by a line drawn from about an inch on either side of the umbilicus to the middle of the space between the symphysis pubis and the crest of the ilium. Its relations to neighbouring parts are as follows:—The peritoneum lies in front of it, separated from it only by a subperitoneal layer of loose fascia, in which the artery and vein lie, which varies much in consistence and amount, and which occasionally gives a good deal of trouble in the operation of ligature. Near its origin it is sometimes crossed by the ureter, and near its termination the genito-crural nerve lies on it. The spermatic vessels cross it, and occasionally a quantity of subperitoneal fat marks its course. *Externally.*—The fascia-iliaca and some fibres of the psoas muscle separate it from the anterior crural nerve, which lies outside of the vessel, and at a somewhat deeper level, hidden amid the fibres of psoas and iliacus. Internally.—The external iliac vein lies on the same plane, and to the inner side of the artery, at Poupart's ligament, on both sides of the body. As we trace it upwards we find that on the left side it lies internal to the artery in its whole course, while on the right side it becomes posterior to the artery as it approaches the bifurcation of the common iliac. Lastly, just before the vessel reaches Poupart, the circumflex iliac vein crosses it from within outwards.

Branches.—The two large branches to the wall of the abdomen, the epigastric and the circumflex iliac, rise a few lines above Poupart's ligament. Their position is unfortunately apt to vary upwards, to the extent of an inch and a half or even two inches, and they are important, as, besides being liable to be cut during the operation, their position very materially modifies the prognosis, as, if too high up, they interfere with the proper formation of the coagulum.

Operation.—Various plans of incision through the skin have been recommended by various operators, the chief difference being with regard to the part of the artery aimed at; the plan known as that of Mr. Abernethy, with various modifications, being intended to expose the artery pretty high up, and enable the surgeon to reach it from above; while the method going by the name of Sir Astley Cooper's exposes the lower part of the artery, and enables the surgeon to reach it from below. Though the latter is in some respects easier, the former method is generally to be preferred, being further from the seat of disease, and especially more out of the way of the epigastric and circumflex arteries.

The higher operation (Abernethy's modified).—An incision must be made through the skin about four inches in length, but longer in proportion to the amount of subcutaneous fat, and the depth of the pelvis, extending from a point one inch to the inside of the anterior superior spine of the ilium, to a point half an inch above the middle line of Poupart's ligament. It must be slightly curved, with its convexity looking outwards and downwards.[3]

The subcutaneous cellular tissue and the tendon of the external oblique may then be divided freely in the same line. Then at some one point or other (generally easiest below), the internal oblique and transversalis muscles must be cautiously scraped through with the aid of the forceps, till the transversalis fascia is reached; they may then be freely divided by a probe-pointed bistoury (guarded by the finger pushed up below the muscles) to the required extent. The muscles being held aside by flat copper spatulæ, the fascia transversalis must be carefully scratched through near the crest of the ilium, and thus the operator will be enabled to push the peritoneum inwards, and by the forefinger will easily recognise the pulsation of the artery lying on the soft brim of the pelvis.

A branch of the circumflex iliac artery will very likely be cut in dissecting through the muscles, and must be secured, as also any branches of the epigastric which may be divided in the incisions through the abdominal wall (ut supra, p. 5).

The operator should then, by pressing the peritoneum and its contents gently inwards, endeavour to see the vessel; if, from the depth of the pelvis, this cannot be done, the sense of touch will be in most cases sufficient to enable him to isolate the artery by the point of his finger-nail, or by the blunt aneurism-needle, from the vein. The ligature should be passed from the inner side to avoid including the vein, and thus there will be less chance of wounding the peritoneum from the convexity of the needle being applied to it. If possible, the genito-crural nerve should not be included in the ligature, but probably such an accident would do no great harm.

It is of much more consequence to avoid injuring the peritoneum. This is sometimes very difficult, from the adhesions which are set up between the peritoneum, the artery, and especially the aneurism, as the result of pressure and inflammation. The accident of wounding the peritoneum has happened to Keate, Tait, Post, and others, and in some cases with perfect impunity. However, the peritoneum should be displaced as little as possible from its cellular

---

[3] The line 3 in Plate I. shows the direction required. It will not be necessary to carry the incision so far up for the external as for the common iliac.

connections, as such displacement increases the risk of diffuse inflammation of that membrane; and the vessel itself should be raised and disturbed as little as possible, lest destruction of the vasa vasorum cause ulceration of the weak coats and secondary hæmorrhage.

The operation from below (Plate I. fig. 4), Sir Astley Cooper's, is thus described by Mr. Hodgson:[4]—"A semilunar incision is made through the integuments in the direction of the fibres of the aponeurosis of the external oblique muscle. One extremity of the incision will be situated near the spine of the ilium; the other will terminate a little above the inner margin of the abdominal ring. The aponeurosis of the external oblique muscles will be exposed, and is to be divided throughout the extent, and in the direction of the external wound. The flap which is thus formed being raised, the spermatic cord will be seen passing under the margin of the internal oblique and transverse muscles. The opening in the fascia which lines the transverse muscle through which the spermatic cord passes, is situated in the mid space between the anterior superior spine of the ilium and the symphysis pubis. The epigastric artery runs precisely along the inner margin of this opening, beneath which the external iliac artery is situated. If the finger therefore be passed under the spermatic cord through this opening in the fascia, it will come in immediate contact with the artery which lies on the outside of the external iliac vein. The artery and vein are connected by dense cellular tissue, which must be separated to allow of the ligature being passed round the former."

In comparing the two methods of operating, we find that while the latter is in some respects easier, and the vessel in it lies more superficial, it has certain disadvantages which more than counterbalance its advantages. Thus, first, the epigastric artery is very likely to be wounded. It may be said, Well, if so, the ends can be tied; but this tying is sometimes very difficult; and, as shown in Dupuytren's case of this accident, involves considerable interference with the peritoneum, and a possibly fatal peritonitis. Besides this, by cutting the epigastric you destroy an important agent which would have carried on the anastomosing circulation, and thus greatly increase the risk of gangrene. By this method, also, the artery is exposed too near to the seat of disease; and if found to be enlarged and involved in the aneurism, considerable difficulty may be experienced in reaching the upper part of the vessel. Again, ligature of the lower third or half of the vessel, which this method implies, is dangerous from the occasional high origin of the circumflex or epigastric, or both, rendering the formation of a clot much more difficult, and secondary hæmorrhage much more likely.

The circumflex iliac vein must also be remembered, as it crosses

---

4 On the Arteries and Veins, p. 421.

7

the artery from within outwards in the lower end of it, just before it goes under Poupart's ligament.

However, the method may occasionally vary with the individual case. In every case of ligature of the great vessels of the abdomen, the bowels should be carefully evacuated before the operation, and the bladder emptied. A properly managed position, with the shoulders raised and the knees semiflexed, will greatly facilitate the gaining access to the vessel.

In sewing up the wounds in the abdominal walls, advantage will be gained by putting in a certain number of stitches so deeply as to include the whole thickness of the muscles, and in the intervals between these deep ones to insert others less deeply, so as accurately to approximate the edges of the skin. This will both facilitate union and also render the occurrence of hernia less probable. This latter accident did occur in a case, otherwise successful, in which Mr. Kirby tied the external iliac.

Both external iliacs have been tied in the same patient with success, on at least two occasions, once by Arendt, with an interval of only eight days between the operations; and a second time by Tait, at an interval of rather more than eleven months.

This operation is in the great majority of cases performed for femoral aneurism, and naturally secondary hæmorrhage is a too frequent result. Wounds of these great vessels generally result in so rapid death from hæmorrhage as to give no time for surgical interference. One case, however, is recorded,[5] in which the external iliac was cut in a lad of seventeen by an accidental stab, and in which Drs. Layraud and Durand, who were almost instantly on the spot, succeeded in stopping the bleeding by compresses, till Velpeau arrived, who tied the vessel above with perfect success.

Of the first twenty-two cases collected by Hodgson, fifteen recovered—a mortality of 31.81 per cent.; and of 153 in Norris's collection, including Cutter's cases, forty-seven died—a mortality of only 32.5 per cent.,—a very satisfactory result, considering the size of the vessel and the importance of its relations.

Ligature of Gluteal.—This vessel, though one of the branches of the internal iliac, approaches the surface so nearly as to be occasionally wounded. It is also, though very rarely, the subject of spontaneous aneurism. The principle of treatment and the operation to be selected in any given case, depends upon its origin, whether traumatic or spontaneous. For if traumatic, the wound must almost necessarily be accessible from the outside; the neighbouring part of the artery is probably healthy, and hence the case can be treated by the old operation, slitting up the tumour, and tying the vessel above and below the wound. When the aneurism is spontaneous, there is no guide to tell

---

[5] Cyclopædia of Practical Surgery, vol. i. p. 277.

us where the aneurism may have first originated; it may be that it is high up in the pelvis, and that the visible tumour is only its expansion in the direction of least resistance, or the coats of the vessel may be extensively diseased. The only chance is ligature of the internal iliac.

1. The old operation, or ligature of the gluteal artery in the hip.

Anatomical Note.—The gluteal is the largest branch of the internal iliac, and leaves the pelvis by the great sacro-sciatic notch just at the upper edge of the pyriformis muscle. After a very short course, it divides into superficial and deep branches opposite the posterior margin of the glutens minimus, between it and the pyriformis muscles.

Very precise rules have been given to enable the operator to hit on the exact spot where the artery leaves the pelvis. These, though perhaps interesting anatomically, are quite useless in a surgical point of view, for the only reasons which could possibly induce a surgeon to cut down upon the gluteal in the living body, are the existence either of a wound of the vessel or an aneurism. In the first the flow of blood, in the second the tumour, would give sufficient guidance.

In cases of traumatic aneurism the operation should be something like the following:—A free incision should be made into the tumour, dividing it in its long direction; the contents should be rapidly scooped out, and a finger placed on the bleeding point, just at the upper corner of the sciatic notch. This will at once stop the hæmorrhage till the vessel can be secured. This sounds easy enough, and has been done several times with success. Thus, John Bell, by an incision two feet long, as he tells us in his hyperbolical language, was enabled to tie the vessel in the case of the leech-gatherer who had punctured the artery by a pair of long scissors. Carmichael of Dublin used a smaller incision, removed one or two pounds of clots, and tied the vessel, in a case of wound by a penknife.[6]

Now, though both of these cases were eventually successful, both patients lost during the operation a very large quantity of blood; John Bell's especially could not be removed from the operating-table for a considerable time after the operation. The period at which the great loss of blood took place was the interval after the incision was made, and before the artery was exposed to view, i.e. the interval in which the surgeon was busy dislodging the clots from the cellular membrane, the sac of the false aneurism. The procedure devised by Mr. Syme to obviate this difficulty, and which was put in practice by him in several very trying cases, is best given in his own terse description of an operation in a case of traumatic gluteal aneurism:—

"The patient having been rendered unconscious, and placed on his right side, I thrust a bistoury into the tumour, over the situation of the gluteal artery, and introduced my finger so as to prevent the blood from flowing, except by occasional gushes, which showed what would

---

[6] John Bell's Prin. of Surg., vol. i. 421; Dublin Jour., vol. iv. 321.

have been the effect of neglecting this precaution, while I searched for the vessel. Finding it impossible to accomplish the object in this way, I enlarged the wound by degrees sufficiently for the introduction of my fingers in succession, until the whole hand was admitted into the cavity, of which the orifice was still so small as to embrace the wrist with a tightness that prevented any continuous hæmorrhage. Being now able to explore the state of matters satisfactorily, I found that there was a large mass of dense fibrinous coagulum firmly impacted into the sciatic notch; and, not without using considerable force, succeeded in disengaging the whole of this obstacle to reaching the artery, which would have proved very serious if it had been allowed to exist after the sac was laid open. The compact mass, which was afterwards found to be not less than a pound in weight, having been thus detached, so that it moved freely in the fluid contents of the sac, and the gentleman who assisted me being prepared for the next step of the process, I ran my knife rapidly through the whole extent of the tumour, turned out all that was within it, and had the bleeding orifice instantly under subjection by the pressure of a finger. Nothing then remained but to pass a double thread under the vessel, and tie it on both sides of the aperture."

The bleeding in this case was thus rendered comparatively trifling, and the patient made a speedy and complete recovery. He returned home within six weeks after the operation.[7]

2. In one case, at least, the gluteal artery has been tied with success (for traumatic aneurism) just where it leaves the pelvis, without the tumour being opened. This was in the practice of Professor Campbell of Montreal. The operation was a very difficult one, and while possible only in cases seen very early, and where the tumour is very small, does not appear to have any advantage over the old method.

Cases of spontaneous aneurism of the gluteal artery should be treated by ligature of the internal iliac. Steven's and Syme's cases of ligature of the internal iliac were of this nature.

Manuals of operative surgery occasionally devote pages to the description of special operations for the ligature of such arteries as the sciatic, epigastric, circumflex ilii, and pudic. They do not require ligature, except in cases of wound either of the vessels themselves or their branches; and, according to the modern principles of surgery in such cases, the ligature should be applied to the bleeding point, rather than to the vessel at a distance above it.

Ligature of Femoral.—Under this head we practically mean cases of ligature of the superficial femoral, for the common femoral, or (as called by some anatomists) the femoral, before the profunda is given off, very rarely requires to be tied. If it is wounded, of course the bleeding point must be sought, and the artery tied above and below it,

---

[7] Observations in Clinical Surgery, Syme, pp. 171-3.

but if an aneurism on the superficial femoral renders ligature of that trunk impossible, experience teaches that ligature of the external iliac gives better results than ligature of the common femoral. Erichsen asserts that out of twelve cases in which the common femoral has been tied, only three have succeeded, the others dying from secondary hæmorrhage. The experience of the Dublin surgeons, Porter, Smyly, and Macnamara, has been more satisfactory, as in eight cases of this operation six were successful.[8] A ninth case was unsuccessful. Reasons to explain the danger are not far to seek, for the numerous small muscular branches, along with the superficial epigastric, circumflex, and pudic trunks, reduce the chances of a good coagulum in the common femoral to a minimum, even without taking into consideration the shortness of the trunk before the great profunda femoris is given off. For the common femoral artery is only from one to two inches in length, and if there are some rare cases in which it is a little later in its bifurcation, there are others in which it divides nearer to Poupart's ligament.

The superficial femoral is the name given to the main trunk between the origin of the profunda, and the point at which, passing through the tendon of the adductor magnus, it receives the name of popliteal. During this long course it gives off no branch large enough or regular enough to receive a name, except one, the anastomotica magna, which rises in Hunter's canal, close to the end of the vessel, so in that respect it is peculiarly suitable for the application of a ligature. Again, in the upper part of its course, it is superficial, being covered only by skin and fascia. A short notice of its most important anatomical relations is necessary.

For the first two inches or two inches and a half of its separate existence, the superficial femoral lies in Scarpa's triangle, covered, as we said, only by skin and fascia. This triangle is formed by the sartorius and adductor longus muscles which meet at its apex, and by Poupart's ligament, which defines its base. The artery lies almost exactly in the centre of the space, and at the apex is covered by the sartorius muscle. The spot where it goes under the sartorius is the one selected for the application of the ligature. The femoral vein lies to the inner side of the femoral artery in this triangle, but their mutual relations vary with the portion of the limb; for, on the level of Poupart's ligament, the artery and vein lie side by side on the same plane, but in different compartments of their sheath; as the artery dives below the sartorius, the vein is still on the inside, but on a plane slightly posterior; while, by the time they reach Hunter's canal, the vein has got completely behind the artery. The separate compartments of the sheath in which the vessels lie are much less marked as the vessels go down the limb, the septum between the artery and the vein being in most cases very ill

---

[8] Brit. Med. Jour. 1867, Oct. 5.

marked, even at the level where the ligature is applied. The anterior crural nerve, which on the level of Poupart's ligament lay outside of the artery and on a plane somewhat posterior, has divided into numerous branches before it reaches the point of ligature. One of its branches requires to be mentioned, and may sometimes be noticed and avoided during the operation, namely the internal saphenous nerve, which, first lying external to the artery, crosses it in front, reaching its inner side just before it enters Hunter's canal, where it leaves the vessel accompanying the anastomotica magna branch.

Operation of Ligature of the Femoral—Scarpa's Space.—The patient being placed on his back, and being brought very thoroughly under chloroform, the knee of the affected limb should be bent at an angle of about 120°, and supported on a pillow. Having previously ascertained the angle of junction of the sartorius and adductor, the surgeon should make an incision (Plate I. fig. 5) just over the pulsations of the vessel, in the middle line of the space, having its lower end quite over the sartorius muscle, and its upper one, at a distance from two and a half to three and a half inches, varying according to the amount of fat and muscle. The saphena vein can generally be recognised, and is almost always safe out of the way of this incision at its inner side.

The first incision should divide the skin, superficial fascia, and fat, quite down to the fascia lata. The edges of the wound being held apart, the fascia should be carefully divided, and the sartorius exposed; its fibres can generally be easily enough recognised by their oblique direction; once recognised, the fascia should be dissected from it till its inner edge be gained, the corner of which should then be turned so that it may be held outwards by an assistant with a blunt hook. The sheath of the vessels is now exposed, and after having thoroughly satisfied himself of the position of the artery by the pulsation, the surgeon should carefully raise a portion of the sheath with the dissecting forceps, and open it freely enough to allow the coats of the artery to be distinctly seen. If the parts are deep, as in a fat or muscular patient, great advantage will be gained by seizing one edge of the sheath by a pair of spring forceps, and committing it to the care of an assistant, while the operator holds the other in his dissecting forceps; there is thus no fear of losing the orifice of the sheath, which without this precaution may easily happen, from the parts being confused with blood, or the position altered by movements of the patient. Now comes the stage of the operation on which, more than on anything else, success or failure depends. A small portion of the vessel must be cleaned for the reception of the ligature, and it must be thoroughly cleaned, so that the needle may be passed round it without bruising of the coats, or rupture of an unnecessary number of the vasa vasorum by rough attempts to force a passage for it. Hence all compromises, such as blunted instruments, silver knives, and the like, are dangerous, for in trying to avoid the Scylla of wounding the artery, they fall into the

12

Charybdis, on the one hand, of isolating too much of the vessel and causing gangrene from want of vascular supply, or, on the other, expose the vein to the danger of injury by the aneurism-needle in their attempts to force it round an uncleaned vessel.

The needle should in most cases be passed from the inner side, care being taken to avoid including the vein which is on the inner side and behind the vessel; the internal saphenous nerve, if seen, should be avoided. The needle must not be passed quite round the vessel raising it up, still less must the vessel be held up on the needle, as used to be done, as if the surgeon was surprised at his own success, but the needle should be passed just far enough to expose the end of the ligature, which must be seized by forceps and cautiously drawn through. It must then be tied very firmly and secured with a reef knot.

The edges of the wound must be brought into accurate apposition, and secured by one or two stitches. If antiseptics are used, drainage should be provided for.

From the very fact that ligature of the superficial femoral is a remarkably successful operation in causing consolidation of the aneurism and a rapid cure, there is also a corresponding danger that the limb be not sufficiently supplied with blood at first. The limb may very possibly become cold, and remain so for some hours at least after the operation. To avoid this as far as possible, it should be wrapped in cotton wadding, and very great care should be taken that it be not over-stimulated by hot applications, friction, or the like, any of which measures might very likely excite reaction, which would result in gangrene.

Complete rest of the limb and of the whole body must be enjoined; the food must be nourishing and in moderate quantity. The chief danger is from gangrene of the limb, which is especially apt to result when the vein is wounded, or even too much handled during the operation.

When properly performed, and in suitable cases, the operation is very successful. Mr. Syme tied this artery for aneurism thirty-seven times, and of these every one recovered. The statistics of Norris and Porta, who collected all the cases in which ligature of the femoral had been employed for any cause, show a mortality of somewhat less than one in four. Rabe's table up to 1869 with the additional cases collected by Mr. Barwell to 1880 gives 297 cases with 53 deaths.[9] Mr. Hutchinson's table, again, of fifty cases collected from the records of Metropolitan Hospitals, shows the very startling result of sixteen deaths out of the fifty cases, or a mortality, in round numbers, of one-third.

Certain anomalies have been observed in the distribution of the femoral vessels, of some importance as affecting the possibility of

[9] International Encyclopædia of Surgery, vol. iii. p. 466.

applying, and the result of, ligature; such as—1. A high division of the branches which afterwards become posterior tibial and peroneal. 2. A double superficial femoral, both branches of which may unite and form the popliteal, as in Sir Charles Bell's well-known case. 3. Absence of the artery altogether, as in Manec's case, where the popliteal was a continuation of an immensely enlarged sciatic.

In such a case the absence of pulsation in front, and the presence of increased pulsation behind the limb, ought to prevent any fruitless attempt at search.

Ligature of the Superficial Femoral below the Sartorius Muscle.— This operation, though once common in France, and though the one recommended by Hunter himself, is now comparatively little used in this country; and rightly so; for while it has no advantage over the upper position, it is at once nearer the seat of disease, and the vessel is more deeply buried under muscles, and has a more distinct fibrous sheath, which requires division.

It is, however, by no means a difficult operation, and is thus performed:—

The limb being laid as before on the outside, and slightly bent, the skin shaved and the pulsation of the artery detected, an incision (Plate I. fig. 6) must be made from the lower edge of the sartorius muscle just as it crosses the vessel, along the course of the vessel, avoiding if possible the internal saphena vein.

The sartorius when exposed must be drawn inwards. The fibrous canal filling the interspace between the abductor magnus and vastus internus is then recognised, and must be fairly opened; the artery is now seen lying in it, and over the vein which is posterior to it, but projects slightly on its outer side; the internal saphenous nerve is lying on the artery. The needle is best passed from without inwards so as to avoid the vein. The anastomotica magna is sometimes a large trunk, and has been mistaken for the femoral in this situation, and tied instead of it.

LIGATURE OF THE POPLITEAL.—This operation is now hardly ever performed for aneurism, ligature of the superficial femoral having quite superseded it, and it is very rarely required for wounds, from the manner in which the vessel is protected by its position.

Before the invention of the Hunterian principle of ligature at a distance, the old operation for popliteal aneurism consisted in cutting into the space, clearing out the contents of the aneurismal sac, and tying both ends of the vessel; from the depth of parts and the close connection of the popliteal vein, this operation was very rarely successful, and is now quite given up. If the vessel is wounded the bleeding point is the object to be aimed at, and is generally sufficient guide.

In cases of hæmorrhage for suppuration of an aneurismal sac, it might possibly be advisable, and there are certain cases of rupture of

14

the artery, without the existence of an external wound, in which attempts have been made to save the limb by tying the vessel.[10] From the complexity of the parts, the numerous tendons, veins, and nerves crowded together in a narrow hollow, and chiefly from the great depth at which the artery lies, any attempt at ligature is very difficult. It is least so at the lower angle of the space, where, between the heads of the gastrocnemius, the vessel comes more to the surface, but is still overlapped by muscle.

Operation.—The patient lying on his face, a straight incision (Plate III. fig. 1), at least four inches in length, should be made over the artery, and thus nearer the inner than the outer hamstring; a strong fibrous aponeurosis will require division after the skin and superficial fascia are cut through, the limb is then to be flexed, and the tendons drawn aside with strong retractors; fat and lymphatic glands must next be dissected through, and then the vein and artery, lying on a sort of sheath of condensed cellular tissue, are seen, the vein lying above the artery and obscuring it. The vein must be drawn to the outside, and the thread passed round the artery, which lies close to the bone, on the ligamentum posticum of Winslowe.

It is a very difficult subject to decide what operations should be described in a work of this character, on the vessels of the leg and foot. A very large number of distinct methods of operations on the various parts of the three chief arteries of the leg have been described by surgeons and anatomists, but specially by the latter.

The fact is, however, that these complicated procedures are rarely required, for aneurisms of the arteries of the leg and foot are almost unknown, while in cases of wound of the vessel, or rupture resulting in traumatic aneurism, the proper treatment is not to tie the vessel higher up, but by dilating the wound and clearing out the clots, if required, to secure the bleeding point, and tie the vessel above and below.

Again, a wound of the sole of the foot often gives rise to very severe and persistent hæmorrhage, while the fasciæ and complicated tendons render ligature of the vessel at the spot very difficult; yet ligature of either the anterior or posterior tibial would probably be insufficient; and to tie both these vessels, with possibly the peroneal and interosseous as well, would be a much more severe and dangerous procedure than ligature of the superficial femoral; while probably careful plugging of the wound, combined with flexion of the knee, will be found to stop the hæmorrhage sooner than either of the more formidable methods.

A competent knowledge of the anatomy of the part, and of the ordinary methods of checking hæmorrhage, such as ligatures, graduated compresses, and styptics, aided by position, specially flexion

---

[10] Poland, Guy's Hosp. Report, ser. iii. vol. vi.

of the knee after Mr. Ernest Hart's method, will suffice to enable the surgeon to check any hæmorrhage of the foot or leg, without it being necessary to burden the memory with the three positions in which to tie the peroneal, or the various methods, more or less bloody and tedious, by which the posterior tibial in its upper third may be secured.

NOTE.—While, as a matter of surgical principle to guide our practice on the living, I still hold very strongly the opinions here expressed against special operations for ligature of the arteries of the leg, and allow the sentences to stand as in the first edition of this work, I insert in a note a brief description of the more important ones, in deference to the advice of friends and the urgent request of pupils, as these operations are used by Examining Boards as tests of the operative dexterity of candidates:—

1. ANTERIOR TIBIAL ARTERY IN LOWER HALF OF LEG.—Anatomical Note.—This vessel is related on its tibial side to the tibialis anticus, and on its fibular, to the extensor longus digitorum above, and the extensor pollicis below. The anterior tibial nerve lies first on its outer side, then crosses the artery, and eventually reaches its inner side near the foot. Operation.—An incision, at least three inches long, parallel with the outer edge of the tibia, and about three-quarters of an inch from it, exposes the deep fascia. This being divided, the outer edge of the tibialis anticus must be found, and will be the guide to the artery, which, surrounded by its venæ comites, lies very deeply between the muscles.

2. POSTERIOR TIBIAL.—A. In middle third of leg. Here the artery is separated from the inner border of the tibia, by the flexor longus digitorum, and is covered by the soleus. *Operation.*—An incision at least four inches long, along the inner margin of the tibia, exposes the edge of the gastroenemius; then divide the tendinous attachment, then expose the soleus, and divide its attachment also; the deep fascia will then be seen; slit it up, and the vessel will be found about an inch internal to the edge of the bone. The nerve is there just crossing it.

Guthrie's, or the direct operation, has the very high authority of the late Professor Spence in its favour. An incision through skin and fascia in the middle of the back of the leg allows the two heads of the gastrocnemius to be separated to the same extent. The soleus is then to be scraped through in same direction, and its deep aponeurotic surface carefully slit up. The artery and vein are then easily seen.

B. In lower third of leg.—This is an easier and more scientific operation, as it does not involve the division of great tendons. An incision midway between the internal malleolus and the tendo Achillis, parallel with both, will expose the very deep and strong fascia in which the tendons lie. The artery, with its

16

venæ comites, occupies a central position, having the tendons of the tibialis posticus and flexor communis in front between it and the internal malleolus, and the posterior tibial nerve behind it, while the flexor longus pollicis lies still nearer the tendo Achillis.

Table illustrating anastomotic circulation after ligature of arteries of lower limb.

1. AORTA.—Epigastric and mammary of both sides. Hæmorrhoidal and spermatic, with branches of pudic both deep and superficial.

2. COMMON ILIAC.—Internal iliac and branches, with those of the other side, along with the following:—

3. EXTERNAL ILIAC.—Internal mammary and deep epigastric.

Iliolumbar and lumbar branches of aorta, with deep circumflex ilii.

Pudic from internal iliac, with superficial pudic of common femoral.

Gluteal, sciatic, and obturator, with the circumflex and perforating branches or deep femoral.

4. FEMORAL.—External circumflex, with external articular of popliteal.

Perforating, with branches of gluteal and sciatic.

Profunda branches with anastomotica and articular branches.

Obturator and internal circumflex with anastomotica and superior internal articular.

NOTE.—The importance of the articular branches of the popliteal explain the danger of gangrene after a sudden rupture or increase in size of a popliteal aneurism.

LIGATURE OF THE INNOMINATE.—The performance of this extremely dangerous, in fact almost hopeless operation, is by no means so difficult as might be expected.

The patient lying down with the shoulders raised and head thrown well back, the sternal attachment of the right sterno-mastoid must be very freely exposed. This may be done by an incision (Plate I. fig. 7) along its anterior edge from the upper edge of the sternum, as far as may be necessary; another about the same length along the upper edge of the clavicle, will meet the former at an acute angle, and will include a triangular flap of skin, which must be carefully dissected up. The sternal, and probably a portion of the clavicular attachment of the right sterno-mastoid, must then be cautiously divided. This being done, the sterno-hyoid and sterno-thyroid muscles require division immediately above their sternal attachments.

A dense process of cervical fascia (just becoming thoracic) now covers the vessel, binding it on the right side to the right innominate vein, and on the left maintaining the relation of the innominate artery to the trachea. The inferior thyroid veins lie on this fascia, and must be

17

drawn aside, not cut. The fascia is then to be scraped through very cautiously, exposing the root of the right carotid, which, being traced downwards, will lead to the innominate. The following parts lie in close relation to the vessel at the point of ligature, and must be avoided:—1. The left innominate vein crosses the artery in front from left to right, and must be drawn down. 2. The right innominate vein and right pneumogastric are in close contact with the artery on the right side; to avoid them the aneurism-needle must be entered on the outside (right of the vessel). 3. The apex of the right pleura and the trachea are in close contact behind, requiring the point of the needle to be kept close to the artery in bringing the thread round.

It might have been expected that the sudden arrest of so large a proportion of the vascular supply of the body, so very near the heart, would cause serious, or even fatal symptoms; this, however, is not the case, no serious inconvenience of this sort being experienced; yet hitherto every case has proved fatal, either from secondary hæmorrhage or inflammation of lungs and pleura.

In fifteen well-authenticated, and in three more doubtful cases, the ligature has been applied; all of these died at periods varying from twelve hours (as in Hutin's case), to forty-two days as in Thomson's, and sixty-seven days (Graefe's).[11]

A successful case of ligature of the innominate along with the right carotid and (after secondary hæmorrhage) the right vertebral, in a mulatto aged thirty-two, for a subclavian aneurism, has been put on record by Dr. Smyth of New Orleans, in the American Journal of Medical Science for July 1866.

And here we may also note that Mr. Heath has lately treated a case of innominate aneurism by simultaneous ligature of the third part of the subclavian and the carotid. Both ligatures separated on the eighteenth day, and the tumour was much smaller some months afterwards.[12]

Mr. R. Barwell has reported several most interesting cases in which simultaneous ligature of carotid and subclavian have proved of marked benefit in aortic as well as in innominate aneurisms.[13]

In four cases the operation was attempted, but the operators had to desist before the application of the ligature, in consequence of the diseased state of the arterial coats. Of these, three died, and one (Professor Porter's of Dublin) case recovered, the patient leaving the hospital with the aneurism nearly consolidated.

Dr. Peixotto of Portugal applied a precautionary ligature to the innominate in a case where secondary hæmorrhage occurred from the

[11] Mr. W. Thomson's most interesting paper on this subject is full of information down to the latest date.
[12] Lancet, Jan. 5, 1867.
[13] Lancet, May 1879.

carotid. The ligature was not tightened beyond what was necessary merely to cause flattening of the vessel. The patient made a good recovery.

Professor George Porter of Dublin records an interesting case of subclavian aneurism, in which, after failing to close the axillary artery by acupressure, he applied L'Estrange's compressor to the innominate itself for three days, with temporary benefit. The patient eventually died of hæmorrhage.[14]

For a very full and interesting account of ligatures of vessels in root of neck we may refer to vol. iii. of the 1883 edition of Holmes' Surgery, pp. 119-122.

LIGATURE OF COMMON CAROTID.—Though the anatomical relations of the right and left carotid are different at their origin, they so precisely resemble each other in the whole of that part of their course which is at all amenable to surgical treatment, that one description will suffice for both, and the necessary anatomy will be brought out quite sufficiently in the description of each operation.

From its giving off no collateral branches, the common carotid artery may be tied at any part of its course.

It has been tied successfully at the distance of only three-quarters, or, in one case by Porter, hardly to be imitated, one-eighth of an inch from the innominate, and up to an equal distance from its bifurcation. In choosing the part of the vessel for operation, the operator must be guided by the position of the aneurism, if on the vessel itself, but if the aneurism be distant, as in scalp or orbit, he need have regard to position simply as facilitating the operation.

The easiest position in which to apply the ligature is just above the omohyoid muscle, the vessel being there superficial.

Ligature above Omohyoid.—Using the anterior border of the sterno-mastoid as a guide, but leaving it gradually above to a little nearer the mesial line, an incision (Plate IV. fig. 1), varying in length according to the depth of fat and cellular tissue in the neck, but with its central point opposite the upper border of the cricoid cartilage, must be made through skin, platysma, and superficial fascia. While making the incision the head should be held back, and the face slightly turned to the opposite side; the parts being now relaxed by position, the edges of the wound must be held apart by blunt hooks or copper spatulæ, and the deep fascia carefully divided over the vessel, which will be recognised by the pulsation. It may be noted here that even in thin subjects the sterno-mastoid edge invariably overlaps the vessel, though in many anatomical diagrams it would appear to be in part subcutaneous.

The descendens noni may possibly be seen, but this is by no means invariably the case, crossing the sheath of the vessel very

---

[14] Dublin Quarterly Journal, Nov. 1867.

gradually from without inwards in its progress down the neck. It must be carefully displaced outwards.

The sheath of the vessel is then to be cautiously opened to the extent of about half an inch. The internal jugular vein, possibly much distended, may overlap the artery on its outer side, and will require to be pressed, emptied, and held out of the way. A small portion of the artery being thoroughly separated from the sheath, the aneurism-needle must be passed from without inwards to avoid the vein, and keep as close to the artery as possible to avoid the vagus.

The tendon of the omohyoid muscle, or, in muscular subjects, a portion of its anterior fleshy belly, may be seen crossing the vessel from above downwards and outwards at the lower angle of the wound.

An enlarged lymphatic gland has occasionally given much trouble, by being mistaken for the vessel and cleaned, while the ligature has even been placed on a carefully isolated fasciculus of muscular fibres.

LIGATURE OF CAROTID BELOW THE OMOHYOID.—An incision in precisely the same direction as the former, but at a slightly lower level, is required, but the dissection is rather more difficult. The edge of the sterno-mastoid when exposed must be drawn outwards; the sterno-hyoid and thyroid inwards; the omohyoid upwards; the sheath opened, and the descendens noni or its branches drawn to the tracheal side. The jugular vein and vagus are both at the outer side, and must be avoided, while the inferior thyroid artery and sympathetic nerve both lie behind the vessel, and may be included in the ligature if care be not taken.

Varieties.—Sedillot's Operation.—To secure the artery still lower in the neck: An incision two and a half inches long, from the inner end of the clavicle obliquely upwards and outwards in the interval between the sternal and clavicular attachments of the sterno-mastoid; this divides the superficial textures; the two portions of muscle must then be drawn apart. The internal jugular vein lies in the interval, and must be drawn to the outside before the artery can be seen at all, and it is this that makes this operation very difficult and dangerous, especially on the left side, where the vein is close to the artery, and probably even crossing it from left to right. The thoracic duct is behind.

Malgaigne's modification of the above is an improvement: to expose the external attachment of the muscle, to cut it through and turn it to the outside, as in the operation for ligature of the innominate, then to divide or pull inwards sterno-hyoid and sterno-thyroid, thus exposing the sheath. The needle must be passed from without inwards.

Results.—Pilz has collected 600 cases, of which 43.16 per cent. died. The united tables of Norris and Wood give 188 cases, with a mortality of sixty, or nearly one in three. These tables include cases in

20

which the vessel was tied for wounds, and as a preparatory step in the operation of removal of tumours of the jaw, etc. Later statistics give a very much lessened mortality, due chiefly to the use of animal ligatures.

Of thirty-one cases in which it was tied for pulsating tumours of the orbit, only two died from the operation.[15] Rivington's statistics to a later date give forty-six cases on forty-four patients with six deaths.

Both carotids have been tied in the same patient twenty-five times, at intervals of less than a year; and it is a very remarkable fact that only five of these fifty ligatures proved fatal,—two in which both were tied on the same day, and three in which the operation was performed to arrest hæmorrhage from malignant disease of the face and jaws—from gunshot wound,—and from syphilitic ulceration.

The external carotid, and also most of its principal branches, have been tied for aneurisms, wounds, goitres, enlargement of the tongue, vascular tumours on occiput and other lesions; also as a first stage in the operation of extirpation of the upper jaw, for the purpose of preventing hæmorrhage. However, such operations are rare, and will probably become rarer still, and it is hardly necessary to describe the operations on each seriatim.

Aneurism of the external carotid or branches are rare; if idiopathic, ligature of the common carotid will be found at once easier, not more dangerous, and more effectual than ligature of the branch; if traumatic, the aneurism itself should be attacked, and the bleeding point secured by a double ligature. Wounds are common enough, but if accessible at all, the injured vessel should be tied at the bleeding point; if inaccessible (and under this head we may include wounds of the internal carotid), the common carotid must be tied.

No one would think of trying the superior thyroids for goitre, unless they were so manifestly enlarged, tortuous, and pulsating, as to render the operation so simple (from their superficial position) as to require no special directions; besides this, the cases in which it has been already done have given very little encouragement to repeat it.

As cases may occur in which any diminution of the cerebral supply is contra-indicated, and thus the more difficult ligature of the external carotid may be preferred to the more simple operation on the common trunk, and as the lingual may require ligature near its root, in consequence of obstinate hæmorrhage from the tongue, short directions are given for the performance of both these operations.

1. LIGATURE OF EXTERNAL CAROTID.—Head in same position as for the common carotid. A straight incision parallel with the anterior edge of sterno-mastoid, but about half an inch in front of it, must begin almost at angle of jaw, and extend downwards nearly to the level of the thyroid cartilage. Cautiously divide skin, platysma, and fascia; the lower end of the parotid must be pulled upwards, and the

---

[15] W. Zehender—Monatsbl. für Augenheilkunde. 1868.

veins, which are numerous, cautiously separated. The anterior border of the sterno-mastoid must be pulled backwards, and the digastric and stylo-hyoid forwards and inwards. The superior laryngeal nerve which lies behind the vessel must be avoided.

2. LIGATURE OF LINGUAL.—To secure this vessel either before it becomes concealed by the hyo-glossus, or after it is under the muscle, a curved incision is necessary, following the line of the hyoid bone, and especially of its greater cornu, but a line or two above its upper border. After the skin and platysma are divided, the posterior belly of the digastric must be recognised, which again will guide to the posterior edge of the hyo-glossus. The edge of the sub-maxillary gland may very probably require to be raised out of the way. The artery can then be secured, either before it dips under the hyo-glossus muscle, or after it has done so, by the division of a few of its fibres on a director. Care is needed to avoid injury of the hypo-glossal nerve, which lies above the muscle.

The internal carotid artery occasionally, but very rarely, is the subject of aneurism. It may, like any other artery, be wounded, especially from the fauces. The treatment of either of these lesions is ligature of the common carotid itself, in preference to ligature of the internal carotid. Guthrie's operation for securing the bleeding internal carotid at the injured spot, by dividing and turning up the ramus of the lower jaw, has never been performed in the living body, and is so difficult, dangerous, and unnecessary, as not to merit description.

LIGATURE OF SUBCLAVIAN.—Note.—In consequence of the difference in the origin, and variety in the anatomical relations of the right and left subclavian arteries, in so far at least as their first stage is concerned, it is necessary to give a very brief separate account of each.

Right Subclavian.—The innominate artery divides into the right subclavian and right carotid exactly behind the sterno-clavicular articulation. The right subclavian extends from this point in an arched form across the neck, between the scalene muscles, over the apex of the pleura, till, passing under cover of the clavicle, it changes its name to axillary at the lower end of the first rib. For convenience of description, the artery is divided into three parts, which have very various anatomical relations, and differ from each other much in their amenability to surgical treatment by ligature. The anterior scalenus muscle defines the three parts, the first extending to the inner border of the muscle, the second being concealed by the muscle, and the third reaching from its outer border to the lower border of the first rib.

Branches of the Subclavian.—While the deep relations of pleura, veins, and nerves can be noticed under the head of each operation in detail, one anatomical point must never be forgotten as influencing very much the success of all surgical interference with the subclavian arteries—i.e. the branches given off. To give any chance of success in the application of a ligature to such a large vessel, so near the heart, a large portion of artery free from branches is required, that the clot may be long, firm, and undisturbed. The first part of the subclavian gives off the vertebral, thyroid axis, and internal mammary; the second, the superior intercostal; while the third part has in most cases no branch whatever. In these anatomical differences we find the reason for the almost invariable fatality resulting on any interference with the first and second parts, and the comparative safety of ligature of the third part, without requiring to account for the difference on other grounds, such as depth of part, importance of nervous relations, or nearer proximity to the heart.

The second and third parts of both arteries are so similar to each other, that a separate account is not required for the two sides.

LIGATURE OF RIGHT SUBCLAVIAN.—*First Part.— Operation.*—An incision just at upper edge of sternum and right clavicle, extending from inner edge of left sterno-mastoid transversely to outer border of right sterno-mastoid through skin, platysma, and exposing sterno-mastoid, to be joined at an angle by a second incision, which, two, three, or even four inches long, must extend along inner border of right sterno-mastoid. Flap to be raised upwards and outwards. The sternal attachment of the sterno-mastoid must then be cautiously divided, as also part or the whole of its clavicular attachment, according as room is required. The sterno-hyoid and thyroid muscles will then require similar division. The internal jugular will then be seen very prominent,[16] and will require to be drawn inwards or outwards, according to circumstances. The carotid and right subclavian arteries will then be felt lying close together crossed by the pneumogastric and recurrent nerves, the latter turning behind the subclavian. The nerves must be drawn inwards; the cardiac filaments of the sympathetic will then be observed, and drawn outwards. The subclavian vein lies below, concealed by the clavicle, and will probably not be seen during the operation. The needle should be passed round the artery from below upwards, care being taken not to injure the pleura, which lies beneath and behind the artery.

Results.—Twelve cases, all of which died; ten of hæmorrhage, one of pleurisy and pericarditis, and one from pyæmia. Attempted in one case by Mr. Butcher, but the artery was too much diseased to bear a ligature. The patient died on the fourth day.

LIGATURE OF LEFT SUBCLAVIAN.—*First Part.*—This operation, which has been described by some as impossible, has, I believe, been only once performed on the living body. Operation.— Incisions as for the preceding operation, except being on the opposite side. After the skin, platysma, and muscles have been divided, as already described, the deep cervical fascia requires division close to the inner edge of the scalenus anticus. The artery lies excessively deep, and

---

[16] Butcher, Op. and Cons. Surgery, p. 861.

great difficulty is experienced in avoiding injury to the pleura and the thoracic duct.

Results.—Once performed by Dr. Rodgers of New York; death from hæmorrhage on fifteenth day.

Anatomical Note.—The course of the left subclavian in its first stage is much straighter, as its origin is much deeper, than on the right side. The pneumogastric, phrenic, and cardiac nerves lie parallel to its course; the œsophagus and thoracic duct lie behind it, and to its inner side.

LIGATURE OF SUBCLAVIAN.—*Second Part.*—This very rare operation hardly requires a separate description, as the incisions necessary for ligature of the artery in its third part will, with very slight modifications, be sufficient for the purpose.

It has, however, special elements of danger in it, involved in the unavoidable division, of part at least, or probably the whole, of the scalenus anticus. The phrenic nerve, from its position on that muscle, requires special care to avoid dividing it, and in most cases the internal jugular vein is also in the way. The branches of the thyroid axis, which cross the neck, are quite in the line of the incision. The lowest cord of the brachial plexus lies immediately behind the artery, between it and the middle scalenus. The pleura lies just below it. The subclavian vein is generally quite safe, running in front of the scalenus anticus, and at a lower level.

The presence of the superior intercostal branch adds greatly to the danger of ligature of the vessel in this position, from its interfering with a proper clot.

Results.—Dupuytren[17] performed it successfully for a traumatic axillary aneurism. Auchincloss[18] did it for a large true aneurism, but the patient died sixty-eight and a half hours after the operation. Liston cut through the outer portion of the scalenus with success for an idiopathic aneurism. Thirteen have been collected by Wyeth with four recoveries and nine deaths.

LIGATURE OF SUBCLAVIAN.—*Third Part.*—For this comparatively common operation, various methods of procedure have been suggested and employed.

In the dead body, where the axilla is free from swelling, and in thin patients, the artery in this third stage is tolerably superficial, and can be secured with ease. But in very muscular men, with short necks and well curved clavicles, and specially when the axilla is filled up with an aneurism, and the shoulder cannot be depressed, the operation becomes very difficult.

Operation of Ramsden, Liston, and Syme.—*Position.*—The patient lying on his back with his shoulders supported by pillows, and

---

[17] Leçons Orales, iv. 530.
[18] Ed. Med. and Surg. Journ. vol. xlv.

his head lying back, and drawn to the opposite side; the shoulder of the affected side must be depressed as much as possible.

Incisions.—(Plate I. fig. 8.)—One through skin, superficial fascia, and platysma, along the upper edge of the clavicle, for at least three inches from the anterior edge of the trapezius to the posterior border of the sterno-mastoid, and in muscular subjects freely overlapping the edges of both muscles. Another two inches in length along posterior border of sterno-mastoid meets the first at an angle. On reflecting the chief flap thus made upwards and backwards, the external jugular will be seen, and, if possible, must be drawn to a side; if not, it must be divided, and both ends tied. The lower edge of the posterior belly of the omohyoid must then be sought; this leads at once to the posterior or outer margin of the scalenus anticus. The connection of the deep fascia to that muscle must then be very carefully scraped through, and by tracing the muscle to its insertion to the first rib, the artery is at once reached, lying behind the insertion. The pulsation of the vessel between the forefinger and the first rib will prove a great assistance; yet care is required, lest one of the branches of the brachial plexus be secured instead of the artery. The lowest cord lies very close to the vessel. The subclavian vein is not likely to give much trouble, from its being on a lower level, and (unless very much dilated) nearly concealed by the clavicle. The suprascapular artery is also hidden, but the transverse cervical crosses the very line of incision, and may give trouble, being occasionally much enlarged, so much so as even for a time to have been mistaken for the subclavian itself. If possible, both these branches should be saved, as being important means of carrying on the anastomosis for the future support of the limb.

An absorbent gland is occasionally in the way, and has even been mistaken for the vessel and carefully cleaned. Such may be removed without scruple.

Care must be taken not to injure the pleura, which lies immediately behind and below the vessel at the seat of ligature. Various instrumental devices have been invented for passing the ligature. The simplest seems still to be best, a common aneurism-needle with a considerable curve.

> Other methods of operating.—A single curved incision above the clavicle, with its concavity upwards, of about three or four inches long, with its inner end rather higher than the outer (Green, Fergusson).
>
> A linear transverse incision in the same situation (Velpeau).
>
> A single linear incision perpendicular to the clavicle (Roux).
>
> An arched incision (Plate IV. fig. 2) with its convexity outwards, and its base on the posterior edge of the sterno-

mastoid, from three inches above the clavicle to the clavicular attachment of the muscle (Skey).

Results.—Dr. Wyeth's Tables in 1877 give 251 cases with 134 or 53 per cent. of deaths.

The late Mr. Furner of Brighton reported a most interesting case, in which he tied both subclavian arteries at an interval of two years in the same patient, for axillary aneurisms, with success.

LIGATURE OF AXILLARY.—*Anatomical Note.*—This vessel, the next stage in the continuation of the subclavian downwards, may be defined surgically as extending from the clavicle to the lower border of the teres major. From the depth of the vessel at its upper part, the numerous nerves, and the close proximity of the vein, the surgeon has carefully to study the anatomical relations. It, like the subclavian, is commonly divided into three stages, and, also like the subclavian, these stages are defined by the relations of the artery to a muscle, the pectoralis minor. Surgically we may draw a very close parallel between the two vessels, for we find that in the axillary, as in the subclavian, the first stage is very deep, and very rarely amenable to ligature; the second, still deeper and more rarely attempted, as in both the operation involves division of a deep muscle; while the third stage in each is the one most frequently chosen by the surgeon.

First Stage.—Between the lower edge of the first rib and upper border of the pectoralis minor the vessel is deeply seated, contained in that process of deep fascia called the costo-coracoid membrane, and covered above by skin, platysma, and the clavicular portion of the pectoralis major. It lies on the first intercostal muscle and the upper digitation of the serratus magnus, while the cords of the brachial plexus are on its acromial side, and the axillary vein in close contact with it on its thoracic side, and frequently overlapping the artery.

Operation.—The great desideratum is free access. An incision (Plate I. fig. 9), semilunar in shape, with its convexity downwards, must extend from half an inch outside of the sterno-clavicular articulation to very near the coracoid process, stopping just before it arrives at the edge of the deltoid, in order to avoid injury of the cephalic vein. It must include skin, fascia, and platysma, and the flap must be thrown upwards. The clavicular portion of the pectoralis major must then be divided right across its fibres, which will retract. The arm must then be brought close to the side to relax the pectoralis minor, which must be drawn aside. The artery will then be felt pulsating, but hidden by the costo-coracoid membrane, which acts as its sheath. This must be carefully scratched through, the nerves pulled outwards, the vein avoided and pulled downwards and inwards, and the thread passed round from within outwards. (Manec, Hodgson, and, with slight modification in the incision through the skin, Chamberlaine.)

26

Ligature has been performed in this position by separating the pectoralis and deltoid muscles, without dividing the muscular fibres (Roux, Desault).

To attempt to gain access between the clavicular and sternal portions of pectoralis major, as has been proposed by some, is almost impracticable in the living body, from the position of the vein, to which, rather than to the artery, this incision leads.

LIGATURE OF AXILLARY, *in its second stage*, is not an advisable operation, when it is merely intended to throw a ligature round the artery for an aneurism lower down.

It has been performed at least twice by Delpech, but it is a rude procedure; in his cases, after the muscle was cut, a dive with the finger was made to collect the whole mass of vessels and nerves, and bring them to the surface near the collar-bone; in this position it is said the artery was easily isolated and tied.

In Mr. Syme's operation of cutting into large axillary aneurisms, and tying both ends of the vessel, the pectoralis minor may, indeed generally has, to be divided, and must take its chance without any special notice or precaution, in the sweeping, free incisions required.

LIGATURE OF AXILLARY *in its third stage.*—This is an operation very much more common, more easy of accomplishment, and safer in its results than either of the preceding; the artery in this stage being more superficial, in fact almost subcutaneous.

Operation.—The arm being extended and supinated, an incision (Plate I. fig. 10) two and a half or three inches long, must be made in the base of the axilla over the artery, involving at first skin and superficial fascia only; the deep fascia is then exposed and must be carefully scraped through, avoiding injury of the basilic vein, if (as sometimes occurs) it has not yet dipped through the fascia. The vessel can now be felt; the median nerve which lies over the artery, or slightly to its outer side, must be drawn outwards, and the axillary vein, which lies at the thoracic side, but often overlaps the vessel, must be carefully drawn inwards. The ligature must then be passed from within outwards.

When the patient is very fat or muscular, the coraco-brachialis muscle may be required as a guide to the vessel; but in general its superficial position renders any guide quite unnecessary, even in the dead body.

Anatomical Note.—While in each stage the axillary artery gives off branches, those arising from the third stage are by far the most important, especially the subscapular, which leaves it at the edge of the muscle of the same name. To avoid these the ligature should be applied as low down on the vessel as possible, and, in point of fact, the operation called ligature of the third stage of the axillary is, anatomically speaking, really ligature of the brachial high up, and where there is room at all, there will be the less chance of secondary hæmorrhage, the greater the distance is between the ligature and the great subscapular branch.

Mr. Syme's Operation for Axillary Aneurism.—Description of the operation in his own words:—

"Chloroform being administered, I made an incision along the outer edge of the sterno-mastoid muscle, through the platysma myoides and fascia of the neck, so as to allow a finger to be pushed down to the situation where the subclavian artery issues from under the scalenus anticus and lies upon the first rib. I then opened the tumour, when a tremendous gush of blood showed that the artery was not effectually compressed; but while I plugged the aperture with my hand, Mr. Lister, who assisted me, by a slight movement of his finger, which had been thrust deeply under the upper edge of the tumour, and through the clots contained in it, at length succeeded in getting command of the vessel. I then laid the cavity freely open, and with both hands scooped out nearly seven pounds of coagulated blood, as was ascertained by measurement. The axillary artery appeared to have been torn across, and as the lower orifice still bled freely, I tied it in the first instance. I next cut through the lessor pectoral muscle close up to the clavicle, and holding the upper end of the vessel between my finger and thumb, passed an aneurism-needle, so as to apply a ligature about half an inch above the orifice."[19]

In a similar operation lately performed by the author for traumatic aneurism, the result of a stab, very little blood was lost, though no incision was made above the clavicle. The patient made a good recovery.[20]

LIGATURE OF BRACHIAL.—To arrest hæmorrhage from a wound of the artery itself, no special directions are required, except to enlarge the wound, and secure the vessel above and below the bleeding point. There are, however, rare cases in which for bleeding in the palm (after all other means have failed), or for aneurism lower down the arm, a ligature may be necessary.

Operation.—The biceps muscle, at its inner edge, is the best guide to the position of the incision, or if it be obscured by fat or œdema, a line extending from the axilla, just over the head of the humerus to the middle of the bend of the elbow will define its course. An incision (Plate I., fig. 11) three inches in length, about the middle of the arm (when you have the choice of position), through skin and superficial fascia, will expose the deep fascia, and probably the basilic vein. Drawing the latter aside, cautiously divide the deep fascia. The artery is then exposed, but in close relation to various nerves; of these the ones most likely to come in the way are—1. The median, which lies

[19] Observations in Clinical Surgery, pp. 148, 149.
[20] Edin. Med. Journal, March 1879.

in front of, but a little to the outside of the artery, though in some rare cases it lies behind it; 2. The internal cutaneous; 3. The ulnar, both of which ought to be rather to the inside of the artery. Two brachial veins accompany and wind round the vessel, occasionally interlacing. Pulsation will, in the living body, usually suffice to distinguish the artery from the other textures, and the ligature may be passed from whichever side is most convenient.

> *Note.*—The relation of the median nerve to the vessel varies according to the part of the arm—thus, as low as the insertion of the coraco-brachialis it is to the outer side, as has been described, it then crosses the vessel obliquely, and two inches above the elbow it is on the inner side of the artery. Again, the operator must never forget the possibility of there being a high division of the artery. This occurs, Mr. Quain has shown, perhaps once in every ten or eleven cases, and may necessitate ligature of both trunks.

In those cases (once much more frequent than at present) where an aneurism has formed after a wound of the brachial at the bend of the arm in venesection, the aneurism may be either circumscribed or diffuse.

If circumscribed, it is advised by some surgeons, specially by the late Professor Colles of Dublin, that the brachial should be tied immediately above the tumour. In most cases of circumscribed, and in all such cases of diffuse aneurism, the preferable operation is boldly to lay open the tumour, turn out all the clots, seek for the wound in the artery, and tie the vessel above and below. A tourniquet above, or, better still, a trustworthy assistant, prevents all fear of hæmorrhage, and such a radical operation exposes the limb to far less chance of gangrene than do any attempts at removing or lessening the tumour by pressure (as recommended by Cusack, Tyrrell, Harrison), and is much more certain than a mere ligature above.[21]

LIGATURE OF VESSELS IN FORE-ARM.—Here, as also we found is the case in the leg, it is almost useless to go on giving exact directions as to the method of throwing a ligature round the vessels in all possible situations.

For below the elbow spontaneous aneurism is almost unknown, and even traumatic aneurisms are extremely rare. It is therefore for hæmorrhage only that the vessels are likely to require ligature, and it is a rule in surgery that to enlarge the wound and to apply a ligature above and below the bleeding point is better practice than to apply a ligature at a distance.

In the case of wounds of the palmar arch, it is extremely difficult, and very apt to injure the future usefulness of the hand, thus to seek for

---

[21] See case of recurrence, Fergusson's Practical Surgery 1st ed. p. 222.

the bleeding point under the palmar fascia, and for these, ligatures of radial and ulnar have occasionally been practised. However, as even this has proved ineffectual, and the interosseous has proved sufficient to continue the bleeding, ligature of the brachial at once is preferable to ligature of so many branches in the fore-arm.

The use of graduated compresses, carefully applied, combined with flexion of the elbow over a bandage, will generally prove sufficient to check such hæmorrhage from the palm, without having recourse to either of the above more severe measures.

Note.—As in the lower limb at page 24, and for the same reasons, I here insert a brief account of the methods of tying the ulnar and radial arteries.

1. Ligature of Ulnar.—Only admissible in the lower half of its course. Operation.—Use the tendon of the flexor carpi ulnaris as a guide, and make an incision along its radial edge, at least two inches in length; expose the deep fascia of the arm and then cautiously divide it; then bending the hand, the flexor carpi ulnaris is relaxed, and the artery is found lying pretty deeply between it and the flexor sublimis digitorum. The ulnar nerve lies at its ulnar side, and the venæ comites accompany the artery. In a tolerably muscular arm, the incision will have to be about an inch inside of the ulnar border of the limb.

2. Radial.—This artery lies more superficial than the preceding, and may be tied at any part of its course.

A. Operation in upper part of fore-arm. Here the artery lies in the interval between the supinator longus and the pronator radii teres. In a muscular arm, the edge of the former muscle is the best guide; in a fat one, the incision may be made in a line extending from the centre of the bend of the arm to the inner edge of the styloid process of the radius. The deep fascia must be exposed and opened, and the muscles relaxed and held aside. The radial nerve lies on the radial side of the vessel.

B. Operation in lower half of arm. Here the vessel is more superficial, lying in the groove between the flexor carpi radialis and supinator longus. An incision two inches in length, and parallel with these tendons, easily exposes the artery. The nerve is still on its radial side.

C. Operation at first metacarpal. The artery may be tied easily enough in the triangular space bounded by the extensors of the thumb, on the dorsum of the proximal end of the first metacarpal bone. Skey[22] recommends a transverse,—

---

[22] Operative Surgery, p. 279.

Stephen Smith[23] and others, a longitudinal incision. The author had lately to secure the radial in its lower third, the superficialis volæ, and the radial again in the triangular space, in a case where division of the artery by a transverse cut had caused a large aneurism to form close above the annular ligament.

Table illustrating anastomotic circulation after ligature of arteries of neck and upper limb.

1. Common carotid.

(a) Across middle line: thyroids, linguals, facials, occipitals; also terminal branches of external carotids; also internal carotids by circle of Willis.

(b) Of same side: occipital with vertebral; superior thyroid with inferior thyroid, etc.

2. Subclavian, 3d part.

Suprascapular with dorsal branches of subscapular; posterior scapular with costal and muscular branches of subscapular. Thoracic anastomosis between internal mammary and intercostals, with branches of axillary.

3. Axillary and brachial. Anastomosis varies with the position of the ligature, but is very free between the various muscular branches of these vessels.

---

[23] Surgical Operations, p. 50.

CHAPTER II

AMPUTATIONS

In ordinary surgical language the name Amputation is applied to all cases of removal of limbs, or portions of limbs, by the knife, though in strict accuracy it should be restricted to those cases in which a limb is removed in the continuity of a bone, its removal at a joint being called a Disarticulation.

The briefest outline of a history of amputation would fill a work much larger than the present. I may be allowed in a few sentences to attempt to show the principle on which such a sketch should be written, in describing the three great eras of progress in improvement of the methods of amputating.[24]

I. Prior to the invention, or at least prior to the general introduction, of the ligature and the tourniquet, the great barrier to all improvement in operating was the impossibility of checking hæmorrhage during an operation, and after its conclusion. Many surgeons would not amputate at all, others only through gangrenous parts; others more bold, only at the confines of parts in which gangrene had been artificially induced by tight ligatures.

With the exception of Celsus, who in one place recommends a flap to be dissected up, and the bone thus divided at a higher level, all were in too great a hurry to get the operation completed to think of flaps. Cut through all the parts at the same level with a red-hot knife, if you will, like Fabricius Hildanus; by a single blow with a chisel and mallet, like Scultetus; or by a crushing guillotine, like Purmannus: or by two butchers' chopping-knives fixed in heavy blocks of wood, one fixed, the other falling in a grove, like Botal; and then try to check the bleeding by tying a pig's bladder over the face of the stump, like Hans de Gersdorf; or tying it up in the inside of a hen newly killed; or by plunging it at once into boiling pitch.

We are the less surprised to read of Celsus's description of a flap operation, when we remember that it is almost certain that Celsus was acquainted with the ligature as a means of checking hæmorrhage.[25]

II. A new era was ushered in when, about 1560, Ambrose Paré invented, or re-introduced, the ligature as a means of arresting

---

[24] For details see article "Amputation" in Cooper's Surgical Dictionary, and the short sketch of the history in Mr. Lister's paper in the third volume of Holmes's System of Surgery.

[25] See a most interesting foot-note to Professor Lister's paper on "Amputation," in Holmes's System of Surgery, vol. iii. pp. 52, 53.

hæmorrhage, but not for more than a century after this did the full benefit of his discovery begin to be felt, when the tourniquet was introduced by Morel at Besançon in 1674, and James Young of Plymouth in 1678, and improved by Petit in 1708-10.

Now surgeons had time to look about them during an amputation, and to try to get a good covering for the bone, so that the stump might heal more rapidly and bear pressure better. Great improvements were rapidly made, and any history of these improvements would need to trace two great parallel lines, one the circular method, the other the flap operation.

1. The old method in which the limb was lopped off by one sweep, all the tissues being divided at the same level, might be called the true circular. This, however, was soon improved—

A. By Cheselden and Petit, who invented the double circular incision, in which first the skin and fat were cut and retracted, and then the muscle and bone were divided as high as exposed.

B. By Louis, who improved this by making the first incision include the muscles also, the bone alone being divided at the higher level.

C. By Mynors of Birmingham, who dissected the skin back like the sleeve of a coat, and thus gained more covering.

D. Then comes the great improvement of Alanson, who first cut through skin and fat, and allowing them to retract, next exposed the bone still further up by cutting the muscles obliquely so as to leave the cut end of the bone in the apex of a conical cavity.

E. An easier mode, fulfilling the same indications, is found in the triple incision of Benjamin Bell of Edinburgh, who in 1792 taught that first the skin and fat should be divided and retracted, next the muscles, and lastly the bone.

F. A slight improvement on E, made by Hey of Leeds, who advised that the posterior muscles of the limb should be divided at a lower level than the anterior, to compensate for their greater range of contraction.

2. In the progress of the flap operation fewer stages can be defined. Made by cutting from within outwards, after transfixion of the limb, the flaps varied in shape, size, position, and numbers, from the single posterior one of Verduyn of Amsterdam, to the two equal lateral ones of Vermale, and the equal anterior and posterior ones of the Edinburgh school.

Then came the battle of the schools: flap or circular.

Flap.—Speedy, easy, and less painful; apt to retract, and that unequally.

Circular.—Leaving a smaller wound, but more slow in performance, and apt to leave a central adherent cicatrix.

3. The last era in amputation began after the introduction of anæsthetics. Now speed in amputation is no object, and the surgeon

33

has full time to shape and carve his flaps into the curves most suited for accurate apposition, and suitable relation of the cicatrix to the bone. It has also been brought clearly out that different methods of operating are suitable for different positions, and also that even in the same operation it is possible to unite the advantages of both the flap and the circular method.

In the modified circular, which is best suited for amputation below the knee, in the long anterior flaps of Teale, Spence, and Carden, we have illustrations of the manner in which the advantages of both the flap and circular methods have been secured, without the disadvantages of either. The long anterior flap, not like Teale's to fold upon itself, but like Spence's and Carden's to hang over and shield the end of the bones, and the face of a transversely-cut short posterior flap, seems to be now the typical method for successful amputations. There may be exceptions, as when the anterior skin is more injured than the posterior, or where an anterior flap would demand too great sacrifice of length of limb, but as a rule it will be found the best method for the patient.

Fig. i

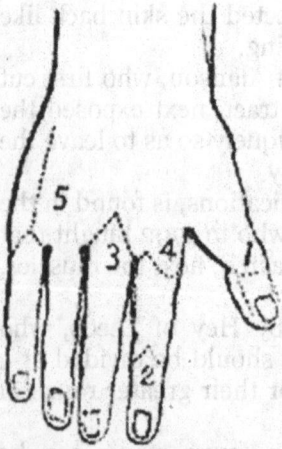

AMPUTATION OF THE UPPER EXTREMITY.—The extreme importance of the human hand, its tactile sensibility, its grasping power, and the irreparable loss sustained by its removal, render the greatest caution necessary, lest we should remove a single digit or portion of one that might be saved. In cases of severe smashing injuries involving the fingers, it is the surgeon's bounden duty not recklessly to amputate the limb with neat flaps at the wrist-joint, but carefully to endeavour to save even a single finger from the wreck, though at the risk of a longer convalescence, or even of a profuse suppuration. While a toe or two, or a small longitudinal segment of the foot, may be comparatively useless, and a good artificial foot, with an ankle-joint stump, certainly preferable, a single finger, provided its motions are tolerably intact, will prove much more valuable to its possessor than the most ingeniously contrived artificial hand.

However, while in cases of extensive smash we endeavour to save anything we can, the case is very much altered when it is only one or two fingers that are injured. Here we find another principle brought into play, and our conservative surgery must be limited by the following consideration. In endeavouring to save a portion of the injured finger or fingers, will the saved portion interfere with the

34

important movements of the uninjured ones? These two principles—1. Generally to save as much as we can; 2. Not to save anything which may be detrimental or in the way,—will guide us in describing the amputations of the upper extremity.

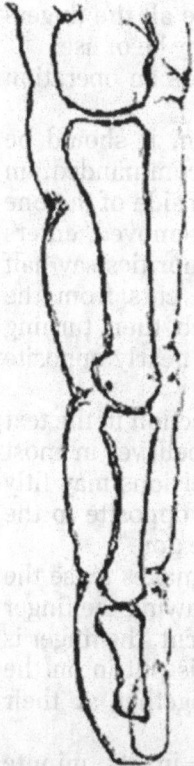

Fig. ii

Amputation of a distal phalanx.—This small operation is not very often required. In cases of whitlow in which the distal phalanx alone has necrosed, removal of the necrosed bone by forceps is generally all that is necessary. In cases of injury, however, in which nail and distal phalanx are both reduced to pulp, it will hasten recovery much to remove the extremity. There is no choice as to flap, the nail preventing an anterior one, so a flap long enough to fold over must be cut from the pulp of the finger in either of two ways (Fig. i. 1):—1. Holding the fragment to be removed in the left hand, and bending the joint, the surgeon makes a transverse cut across the back of the finger, right into and through the joint, cutting a long palmar flap from within outwards as he withdraws the knife.

Note.—Some difficulty is often felt in making the dorsal incision so as exactly and at once to hit the joint; the most common mistake being, that the transverse incision is made too high, and the knife, instead of striking the joint, only saws fruitlessly at the neck of the bone above. To avoid this, the surgeon should take as a guide to the joint, not the well-marked and tempting-looking dorsal fold in the skin, but the palmar one, which exactly corresponds with the joint between the proximal and middle phalanges, and is only about a line above the distal articulation.—(Fig. ii.)

2. Making the long flap by transfixion, it may be held back by an assistant, and the joint cut into.

Amputation through the second phalanx.—If the distal phalanx be so much crushed that a flap cannot be obtained, two short semilunar lateral flaps may be dissected (Fig. i. 2) from the sides of the second phalanx, which may then be divided by the bone-pliers at the spot required.

In cases of injury which do not admit of either of the preceding operations, it is quite possible to amputate either at the first joint, or even through the proximal phalanx. Patients are sometimes anxious for such operations in preference to amputation of the whole finger. The surgeon should, however, never amputate through a finger higher up

35

than the distal end of the second phalanx, unless absolutely compelled by the patient, for the resulting stump, being no longer commanded by the tendons, will prove merely an incumbrance, and may possibly require a secondary operation at no distant date for its removal.

This rule is applicable in cases in which a single finger is injured, and two or three complete ones are left; in cases where all the fingers have been mutilated every morsel should be left, and may be of use.

Amputation of a whole finger.—(Fig. i. 3)—This is an operation of great importance, from its frequency.

If the third or fourth digits require amputation, it should be performed as follows:—The vessels of the arm being commanded, an assistant holds the hand, separating the fingers at each side of the one to be removed. The surgeon holding the finger to be removed, enters the point of a long straight bistoury exactly (some authorities say half an inch) above the metacarpo-phalangeal joint, and cuts from the prominence of the knuckle right into the angle of the web, then, turning inwards there, cuts obliquely into the palm to a point nearly opposite the one at which he set out.

Note.—While most authorities agree with the direction in the text regarding the palmar termination of the incision, I believe, in most cases, it is not necessary to go so far, and that the incisions may fitly meet in the palm at a point midway between a point opposite to the knuckle, and the centre of the well-marked "sulcus of flexion."

He then repeats this incision on the other side, makes tense the ligaments, first at one side and then at the other, by drawing the finger to the opposite side, and cuts them. The tendons being cut, the finger is detached. The vessels being tied, one point of suture is put in on the dorsal aspect, and the fingers on each side tied together at their extremities, with a pad of lint between them.

Modification.—Lisfranc's method is too long in its minute description to give in detail. The principle is to make a semilunar flap at one side (the one opposite the operator's right hand), by cutting from without inwards, then to open the joint from this cut, and, still keeping the edge of the knife close to the head of the phalanx, cutting the other flap from within outwards. This can be very rapidly done, but the last flap is apt to be irregular and deficient, especially in those common cases, in which, after whitlow or the like, the tissues are hard and brawny, and the skin does not play freely.

It is quite unnecessary to remove the head of the metacarpal, either for the sake of appearance, or to render healing more rapid, and its removal weakens the arch of the hand; where the cartilage is eroded by disease, the cartilage-covered portion can be scooped off by a gouge or removed entire by pliers, without interfering with the broad end to which the transverse ligament of the palm is attached. If required either for injury or disease, the metacarpal head may be easily removed by a single straight incision from the knuckle upwards, as far as the point at which it may be deemed necessary to saw it through, or better still, divide it with the bone-pliers. This incision should be made as a first step in the first incision for amputation of the finger, and the finger should not be disarticulated, but kept on, to aid by its leverage in separating the metacarpal head.

Amputation of the index or little fingers.—This operation differs from the preceding only in this, that care must be taken to make a good large flap on the free side of each; making the incision, which begins at the knuckle (Fig. i. 4), enclose a well-rounded flap, and not allowing it to enter the palm till it reaches the level of the web between the fingers. The metacarpal heads may here be cut obliquely with the bone-pliers, to prevent undue projection.

Amputation of one or more metacarpals.—These operations may be rendered necessary by disease or injury. If the latter demands their performance, no rules can be given for incisions or flaps, they must just be obtained where and how they can best be got. If for disease, a single dorsal incision (Fig. i. 5) over the bone will allow it to be dissected out of the hand.

N.B.—In no case, except that of the thumb, should any attempt be made to save a finger while its metacarpal is removed. (See Excisions of Bones.)

Amputation of first and fifth metacarpals.—Various special operations have been devised for speedy and elegant removal of these bones. Their disadvantages, etc., are fully detailed under Amputations of the Foot.

The vascularity and consequent vitality of the tissues of the hand and arm sometimes afford very encouraging and satisfactory results in conservative operations.

The following is an instance of what may be accomplished in a young healthy subject.

A. A., æt. 18, ploughman, was harnessing a vicious horse, when it caught his right hand between its teeth, and gave a severe bite. On admission, I found the middle and ring fingers completely separated at the metacarpal joints, but each hanging on by a portion of skin, the middle by the skin on its radial side, the ring by that on its ulnar. The back and the palm were both stripped of skin up to the middle of the third and fourth metacarpal bones, which were exposed, but not fractured. As it was important for him to maintain the transverse arch of the hand intact, I determined to make an attempt to save the metacarpals, and finding that the skin on the radial side of the middle, and ulnar side of the ring fingers, was still warm, and apparently alive, I carefully dissected as long a flap as possible from each, and then folded them down, one at the front, the other at the back of the hand. The flaps survived, and the result was admirable, the patient being able in a very few weeks to guide the plough. The sensation in his new palm and back of the hand is very peculiar, they being still the fingers, so far as nervous supply is concerned.

In amputations involving the metacarpals for injury, it is always important to avoid entering the carpo-metacarpal joint, hence if it can be done it is best to saw through the bones at the required level, rather than disarticulate. This rule should be observed even in those cases in which the thumb alone can be saved, for notwithstanding the isolation of the joint between the first metacarpal and the trapezium, it is very important for the future use of this one digit that the motions both of the wrist and carpal joints should be preserved entire.

No exact rules can be given for the performance of these operations, as the size and positions of the flaps must be determined by the nature of the accident and the amount of skin left uninjured.

In the rare condition where the greater part of the metacarpus is destroyed, and yet carpal joints are uninjured, a most useful artificial band, preserving the movements of the wrist, may be fitted on; and as much as possible should be saved, but in cases of injury, where the carpus is opened and the hand irreparably destroyed, the question arises, Where ought amputation to be performed? To this we answer that there appears no conceivable advantage to be gained by leaving all or any of the carpal bones. If successful, it would result only in the retention of a flapping joint, unless from there being no tendons to act upon it, except the tendon of the flexor carpi ulnaris attached to the pisiform, and there are several risks it would run in the inflammation of all the carpal joints, and the almost certain spread of this inflammation to the bursa underneath the flexor tendons, beyond the annular ligament, and up the arm among the muscles.

AMPUTATION AT THE WRIST-JOINT.—This is an operation by no means frequent, and it has the advantages of preserving a long stump, and retaining the full movements of pronation and supination, in cases where the radio-ulnar joint is sound and uninjured, but in practice it is often found that fibrous adhesions limit to a great extent the motions of the two bones on each other, specially in those cases where the radio-ulnar joint has been diseased or injured.

Another advantage is the extreme ease with which disarticulation may be performed on emergency, no saw being required, and the ordinary bistoury of the pocket-case being quite sufficient for cutting the flaps.

Operation.—By double flap. An incision (Plate IV. fig. 3) on the dorsal surface, extending in a semilunar direction from one styloid process to the other, will define a flap of skin only, which must be raised; the joint must then be opened by a transverse incision, and a long semilunar flap of skin and fascia should be shaped (Plate IV. fig. 4) from the palm. Disarticulation is facilitated by the surgeon forcibly bending the wrist when he makes the transverse cut, and it will be found easier to shape the palmar flap from the outside by dissection, than to do it by transfixion after disarticulation, on account of the prominence of the pisiform on the inner side of the palm.

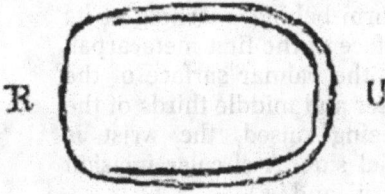

Fig. iii.

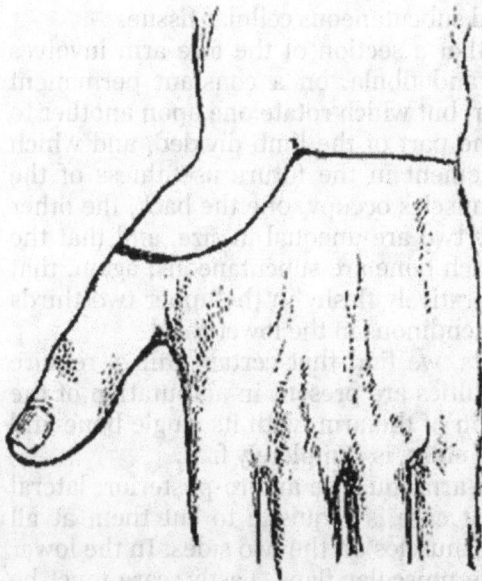

Fig. iv.[26]

In the thin wasted wrists of the aged, or in any case where the skin is very lax, this amputation may be very easily performed by the circular method. While an assistant draws up the skin as much as possible, the surgeon makes an accurate circular incision through the skin, about an inch below the styloid processes, just grazing the thenar and hypothenar eminences. Another circular sweep just above the pisiform and unciform bones divides all the soft textures, after which the joint may be opened, and, if necessary, the styloid processes cut away with saw or pliers.

Amputation by a long single flap, either dorsal or palmar, may be rendered necessary by accident. The palmar one of the two is preferable; indeed, rather than trust for a covering to the thin skin of the back of the hand, with its numerous tendons, it is better to amputate an inch or two higher up through the fore arm.

The following amputation by external flap has been described (so far as I can discover, for the first time) by Dr.

---

[26] Fig. iv. shows dorsal view of incision. Fig. iii. showsface of completed stump; R, radial; U, ulnar.

Dubrueil, in his work on operative Surgery:[27]—"Commencing just below the level of the articulation, while the hand is pronated, the surgeon makes a convex incision, beginning at the junction of the outer and middle thirds of the arm behind, reaching at its summit the middle of the dorsal surface of the first metacarpal, and terminating in front just below the palmar surface of the joint, again at the junction of the outer and middle thirds of the breadth of the arm. This flap being raised, the wrist is disarticulated, beginning at the radial side. A circular incision finishes the cutting of the skin." (Figs. iii. and iv.)

AMPUTATION THROUGH THE FORE-ARM.—The method of operating must, in the fore-arm, depend a good deal upon the part of the arm where you require to amputate, the muscularity of the limb, and the condition of the skin and subcutaneous cellular tissue.

It must be remembered that a section of the fore-arm involves two bones, not, like the tibia and fibula, on a constant permanent relation in position to each other, but which rotate one upon another to an amount which varies with the part of the limb divided, and which rotation is a very important element in the future usefulness of the stump; again, that two sets of muscles occupy, one the back, the other the front of the limb, that these two are unequal in size, and that the outer sides or rather edges of each bone are subcutaneous; again, that these sets of muscles are comparatively fleshy in the upper two-thirds of the limb, and almost entirely tendinous in the lower third.

Remembering these points, we find that certain things require our attention, and certain difficulties are present in amputation of the fore-arm, from which amputation of the arm, with its single bone and copious muscular covering on all sides, is completely free.

Thus our flaps in the fore-arm must be antero-posterior; lateral flaps are an impossibility. Great care is requisite to cut them at all equal, from the inequality of the muscles on the two sides. In the lower third we cannot obtain available muscular flaps. Lastly, care must be taken lest, from the ever-varying relations of the two bones to each other in the varying positions of the limb, the surgeon mistake their position and pass his knife between them.

The next question that arises is, Where are we to operate? In cases where we have a choice, is there here, as in the leg, any "point of election"? No. As a rule in the fore-arm, the surgeon should endeavour to save as much as possible; especially when nearing the middle of the fore-arm, he should try to save the insertion of the pronator teres, so important in its function of pronating the radius.

AMPUTATION IN LOWER THIRD OF THE FORE-ARM.—By two flaps. These antero-posterior flaps must consist of skin only, as the tendons are only in the way, and thus should be made by dissection

---

[27] Manuel d'Opérations chirurgicales.

40

from without.[28] Making the dorsal one first, the surgeon should enter his knife at the palmar edge of the bone that is further from him, and cut a semilunar flap of skin only, finishing the incision quite on the palmar edge of the inner bone. The two ends of this incision must then be united by a similar semilunar flap of skin on the palmar side. The two flaps having been dissected back, he then clears the bones by a circular incision through tendons and muscles, not forgetting to pass the knife between the bones, and retracting all the soft parts, saws through the bones, at least half or probably three-quarters of an inch higher up. It is generally easiest to saw through both bones at once.

Long Dorsal Flap.—Where it is possible from laxity of the soft parts and the wrist not being much destroyed, to get a long flap from the back of the arm after Mr. Teale's method, a very good stump will result. This rule is, "In tracing the long flap a longitudinal line is drawn over the radius, so as to leave the radial vessels for the short flap (Plate II. fig. 1). At a distance equal to half the circumference of the limb, another line parallel to the former is drawn along the ulna. These are then joined at their lower ends, across the dorsal aspect of the wrist or fore-arm, by a transverse line equal in length to half the circumference of the fore-arm. The short flap is marked by a transverse line on the palmar aspect, uniting the long ones at their upper fourth.

"The operator, in forming the long flap, makes the two longitudinal incisions merely through the integuments, but the transverse one is carried directly down to the bones. In dissecting the long flap from below upwards, the tissues of which it is composed must be separated close to the periosteum and interosseous membrane. The short flap is made by a transverse incision through all the structures down to the bones, care being taken to separate the parts upwards close to the periosteum and membrane." The stump must be placed in the prone position, "to allow the long dorsal flap to be the superior when the patient is recumbent, and thus fall over the ends of the bones."[29]

The principal objection to the long dorsal rectangular flap (which makes an excellent covering) is, that unless it can be obtained from over the wrist-joint it requires the bones to be sawn so very high up. This may be avoided, to some extent, by making it shorter and rounded off, as in Carden's Amputation, q.v.

AMPUTATION IN UPPER TWO-THIRDS.—Where the fore-arm is very fat or fleshy, this amputation can be very easily performed by two equal antero-posterior flaps made by transfixion. In most cases, however, from the comparative leanness of the dorsal aspect of the limb, the following method will have the best result. The surgeon must,

---

[28] As the surgeon will find it most convenient to stand on his own right side of the limb to be removed, the knife will be entered on the palmar side of the radius of the right arm, of the ulna of the left.

[29] Teale, On Amputation by Rectangular Flaps, pp. 46-48.

as in the former case, shape a rounded dorsal flap by dissection from without (Plate IV. fig. 5), embracing the whole breadth of the limb down to the palmar edge of both bones. Then at once he transfixes the two points of this dorsal flap, and cuts out an equal one from the anterior aspect of the limb (Plate IV. fig. 6). Dissecting up the dorsal flap he clears the bones at least half an inch above as before, and applies the saw.

> N.B.—This operation should be performed even in cases where only an inch of radius can be retained, as the attachment of the biceps makes a very small stump of fore-arm wonderfully useful.

AMPUTATION AT ELBOW-JOINT.—In cases where it is found impossible to save any portion of the fore-arm, disarticulation at the elbow-joint may be easily performed. This operation was proposed and performed so long ago as the days of Ambrose Paré,[30] was much approved by Dupuytren, Baudens, and Velpeau, had fallen into disuse for a time, but is now again recommended by some excellent surgeons, especially by Gross[31] and Ashhurst,[32] both of Philadelphia.

It is tolerably easy to perform, and does not involve any sawing of bones, but the flaps are apt to be cut too short, unless care be taken, from the manner in which the trochlea projects downwards beyond the line of the condyles, so that if the base of an ordinary-shaped flap be made on a level with the condyles, it will prove insufficient to cover the bone. It may be performed either by the circular method (Velpeau), oval (Baudens), or by a long anterior and short posterior flap (Textor and Dupuytren). Probably the best method is by a long anterior flap when it can be obtained, thus:—The arm being placed in a slightly flexed position, the surgeon transfixes in front of the joint, in a line extending from the level of the external condyle to a point one inch below the internal condyle (Plate IV. fig. 7); the tissue should be held well forward at the moment of transfixion. The flap should be at least two and a half inches deep at its apex, which must be rounded off. The two ends of this flap may then be united behind by a semilunar incision (Plate III. fig. 2), which will separate the radial attachments. The ulna must then be cleared, and the triceps divided at its insertion.

> Modifications.—Dupuytren used to saw through the ulna, leaving the olecranon attached. Velpeau opposed this, but it is again recommended by Gross, who leaves the olecranon, and at the same time improves the shape of the stump by sawing off the "inner trochlea" on a level with the general surface.

AMPUTATION OF THE ARM.—This amputation is best

---

[30] Johnson's folio ed., p. 342.
[31] Gross's Surgery, 6th ed. vol. ii. p. 1103.
[32] International Encyclopædia of Surgery, vol. i. p. 641.

performed by double flap, and is the typical instance which exhibits all the advantages of two equal flaps made by transfixion, without any of the disadvantages of that method. These advantages are, easiness of performance, rapidity, excellent covering for the bone, with as little sacrifice of tissue as is possible, while the fact that the cicatrix is opposite the end of the bone is hardly a disadvantage in the arm (as it certainly is in the leg), as no weight has to be borne on it. When they can be obtained, anterior and posterior flaps are generally considered most satisfactory, but Mr. Spence prefers lateral ones, lest the line of union should be interfered with by the deltoid raising the bone. If the right arm has to be amputated, the operator standing at the inner side raises the anterior muscles with his left hand, and enters the knife just in front of the brachial vessels (Plate I. fig. 12); keeping as close as possible to the bone, he brings out the knife at a point exactly opposite, then with a brisk sawing motion, cuts a semicircular flap, taking care to bring out the knife more suddenly just at the end, in order to cut through the skin as perpendicularly to the arm as possible. The knife is again entered at the same point, carried behind the bone, and brought out at the same angle, and an exactly corresponding flap cut from the other side of the limb, the flaps are then retracted, the bone cleared by circular incision and sawn through as high up as it is exposed. In primary cases, where the muscles are firm and developed, the flaps should be cut a little concave.

Modifications and Varieties.—Teale's method may of course be used here as elsewhere. The internal line of incision (Plate IV. fig. 8) should be made just in front of the brachial vessels. This method requires the amputation to be performed higher up than would otherwise be necessary (from the length of the anterior flap), and this disadvantage is not counterbalanced by any special advantage in the posterior retraction of the cicatrix.

In feeble flabby arms, the true circular operation is very easily performed, and with good results. A circular sweep of the knife is made through the skin alone, which is drawn up by an assistant, while the surgeon separates it from the fascia; another circular cut through fascia and muscles exposes the bone, which must then be cleared and cut through at a still higher level.

AMPUTATION AT THE SHOULDER-JOINT.—This operation, like that at the hip joint, can, from the nature of the joint to be covered, and the abundant soft parts in the normal state of the tissues, be performed on the dead in very various ways, by single, double, or triple flaps, by transfixion or dissection, rapidly or slowly. Hence manuals of operative surgery might collect at least twenty different methods, most

43

of which have some recommendation, and all of which are practicable enough.

When, however, we reflect that in the living body, in cases where amputation at the shoulder-joint is required at all, the severity of the accident, or the urgency of the disease, will, in general, leave no room for selection, we shall see how utterly valueless is any knowledge of mere methods of operating, and of how much greater importance it is that we should be simply thoroughly familiar with the anatomy of the joint.

For example, an accident which necessitates amputation so high up has, in all probability, opened into the joint and destroyed the soft parts on at least one aspect; in such a case the flaps must be cut from the uninjured soft parts only. If an aneurism has rendered amputation through it and through the joint a last resource, the flap must be gained chiefly at least from the outside; a malignant tumour of the humerus will almost certainly prevent any transfixion, and require flaps to be made by dissection, wherever the skin is least likely to be involved. Again, some of the most vaunted and most rapid operations almost require for their success the integrity of the humerus, which has to make itself useful as a lever in disarticulation, while in most cases of accident we are amputating for compound injury of the humerus, almost certainly implying fracture with comminution.

From its proximity to the trunk, hæmorrhage is one of the chief dangers to be apprehended during this operation, especially from the axillary artery. As far as possible to obviate this danger, most plans of operating are based on the principle that the vessels and nerves should be the last tissues to be cut; in some they are not divided till after disarticulation.

While a good assistant, to make pressure on the subclavian above the clavicle, is a most advisable precaution, too much must not be trusted to this pressure above, as the struggles of the patient and the spasmodic movements of the limb, which are so apt to occur under the stimulus of the knife, are apt to render futile the best efforts at compression.

The operator should trust rather to making the incisions in such a manner that the great vessel be not divided till the hand of an assistant, or in default of a suitable one, his own left hand, is able to follow the knife and grasp the flap.

The bleeding from the circumflex, subscapular, and posterior scapular arteries can easily be arrested by a dossil of lint till the great vessel is tied, and they can be secured.

In cases where proper assistants cannot be had, temporary closure of the axillary vessel could easily be made by carrying a strong silver wire or silk ligature completely round the vessel by a curved needle before the incisions are commenced, and by tying this firmly over a pad of lint.

Pressure on the artery above the clavicle is best made by the thumb of a strong assistant, who endeavours to compress it against the first rib; where the parts are deep and muscular, the padded handle of the tourniquet, or of a large door-key, will do as the agent of pressure.

A brief notice of three of the best methods of operating will be quite sufficient to show what should be aimed at in shoulder-joint amputations:—

1. In cases where the surgeon can choose his flaps, the following method will be found the most satisfactory, as resulting in the smallest possible wound, in having less risk of hæmorrhage during the operation than any other method, and in providing excellent flaps.

It is Larrey's method slightly modified.

Operation.—With a moderate-sized amputating knife an incision of about two inches in length, extending through all the tissues down to the bone, should be made from the edge of the acromion process to a point about one inch below the top of the humerus; from this latter point a curved incision, enclosing a semilunar flap, should be made on each side of the limb to the anterior and posterior folds of the axilla respectively (Plate IV. fig. 9, and Plate III. fig. 3). These flaps should then be dissected back, including the muscles and exposing the joint. When thoroughly exposed, the joint must then be opened from above, and the bone separated. One small portion of skin lying above the artery, vein, and nerves still remains to be divided (Plate I. fig. 13). This may be done by an oblique cut from within outwards, in such a direction as to form part of the anterior or internal incision, and with the precaution of having an assistant to command the vessels before they are divided. The resulting wound is almost perfectly ovoid, the flaps come together with great ease in a straight vertical line, which admits of easy and thorough drainage. Union is generally rapid. Larrey's success by this method was very remarkable: ninety out of a hundred cases in military practice were saved, notwithstanding the well-known risks of such operations.

2. As good as the former, and nearly as universally applicable, is the method devised by Professor Spence, and practised by him in nearly every case:—"With a broad strong bistoury I cut down upon the inner aspect of the head of the humerus, immediately external to the coracoid process, and carry the incision down through the clavicular fibres of the deltoid and pectoralis major muscles till I reach the humeral attachment of the latter muscle, which I divide. I then with a gentle curve carry my incision across and fairly through the lower fibres of the deltoid towards, but not through, the posterior border of the axilla. Unless the textures be much torn, I next mark out the line of the lower part of the inner section by carrying an incision through the skin and fat only, from the point where my straight incision terminated, across the inside of the arm to meet the incision at the outer part. This insures accuracy in the line of union, but is not

essential. If the fibres of the deltoid have been thoroughly divided in the line of incision, the flap so marked out, along with the posterior circumflex trunk, which enters its deep surface, can be easily separated from the bone and joint, and drawn upwards and backwards so as to expose the head and tuberosities, by the point of the finger without further use of the knife. The tendinous insertions of the capsular muscles, the long head of the biceps, and the capsule, are next divided by cutting directly upon the tuberosities and head of the bone; and the broad subscapular tendon especially, being very fully exposed by the incision, can be much more easily and completely divided than in the double-flap method. By keeping the large posterior flap out of the way by a broad copper spatula or the fingers of an assistant, and taking care to keep the edge of the knife close to the bone, the trunk of the posterior circumflex is protected. In regard to the axillary vessels, they can either be compressed by an assistant before completing the division of the soft parts on the axillary aspect, or to avoid all risk, the axillary artery may be exposed, tied, and divided between two ligatures so as to allow it to retract before dividing the other textures."[33]

Another, but not so good method of making an external flap, is the following:—(a.) For the right arm.—The patient lying well over on his left side, the surgeon stands to the inside of the arm to be removed. Seizing the deltoid in the left, with the right he passes an amputating knife, seven or eight inches in length, from a point a little nearer the clavicle than the middle space between the acromion and coracoid processes; then, transfixing the base of the deltoid, and just grazing the posterior surface of the humerus, thrusts the knife downwards and backwards till it protrudes at the posterior margin of the axilla. When doing this, it is important that the arm be held outwards and backwards, and even upwards, as far as possible to relax the deltoid; without this it will be impossible to make the flap of the full size. The flap must then be cut of as full length as can be obtained, four or five inches at least. An assistant then holds it upwards, while the surgeon, or (if the arm is very muscular) another assistant, brings the arm forwards well across the patient's chest, thus exposing the posterior aspect of the joint. This may have very possibly been already opened during the transfixion; the attachments of muscles must now be divided, the knife passed behind the head of the bone, which is dislocated forwards, and a suitable flap of the tissues in front cut from within outwards. The assistant is to follow the knife with his finger and compress the vessels.

(b.) If the left shoulder is to be amputated, the patient lying on his right side, the surgeon stands behind him, and raising the elbow of the limb to be removed from the side, and

---

[33] Spence's Surgery, pp. 800, 801.

pulling it slightly backwards, enters the knife at the posterior fold of the axilla (Plate II. fig. 2), and passing the posterior aspect of the head of the humerus, endeavours to protrude it as near the acromion as possible; the flaps must be cut and the rest of the operation performed in the manner we have just described for the other arm.

3. Where the destruction of tissue has been chiefly below the joint, a very good flap may be obtained from above, composed chiefly of the deltoid muscle, and the skin over it. This may be made by transfixion at its base, but is better obtained by dissection from without.

The surgeon cuts (Plate II. figs. 3, 3) in a semilunar direction (with the convexity downwards) from one side of the deltoid to the other, viz., from the root of the acromion to near the coracoid process; he then raises the large flap upwards and throws it back, opens the joint, disarticulates, passes the knife behind the head of the bone, and cuts out without attempting to save any flaps below, in a transverse direction. By this means the artery is still almost the last structure to be divided, and can be secured by a ready assistant. In cases where much injury has been done to the floor of the axilla and wall of chest, the deltoid flap must be made large in proportion, and triangular rather than semilunar in shape.

N.B.—The statistics of amputation at the shoulder-joint bring out some interesting facts: 1. That the primary amputations here are far more successful than secondary ones. Guthrie records nineteen cases of the former out of which only one died, while out of a similar number in which the amputation was secondary, fifteen died. In the Crimea, British surgeons had thirty-nine cases, with thirteen deaths; of thirty-three primary, nine died; and of six secondary, four were fatal.

S.W. Gross's[34] statistics confirm this: of one hundred and seventy-eight primary, forty-six died—25.8 per cent.; ninety-five secondary, sixty-one died—64.2 per cent.

Amputations above the Shoulder-Joint.—Under this head we may group the comparatively rare cases in which, from accident or disease, the removal of portions of the scapula and clavicle, or even the entire bones, is rendered necessary. That it is quite possible to survive such injuries has been frequently shown in cases of accident when the scapula along with the arm has been torn off, and yet the patient recovered.

Encouraged by such cases, Gaetani Bey of Cairo removed the whole of scapula and part of the clavicle in a case where he had amputated at the shoulder for smash. The patient recovered. Heron Watson has had a similar case. Dr. George M'Lellan amputated arm

---

[34] Gross's Surgery, 8vo., 6th ed., vol. ii., p. 1106.

and scapula in a youth of seventeen for an enormous encephaloid tumour. Fifty-one such cases are now on record.

Syme amputated with success the arm along with the scapula and outer half of clavicle, in a case in which he had previously excised the head of the humerus for a tumour.[35]

Gilbert, Mussey, Rigaud, Fergusson, and others have performed similar operations, secondary to amputation at the shoulder-joint, for cases of caries and malignant tumour. It is impossible to give any exact directions for the incisions which must be planned for individual cases, with two chief aims, to avoid hæmorrhage as far as possible, and to leave abundance of skin. In operations on the scapula, it should be freely exposed by large enough incisions. (See Excisions.)

AMPUTATIONS OF LOWER EXTREMITY.—Commencing with the most distal, and gradually working our way upwards, we find that partial amputations of the toes are extremely rare. Only in the case of the great toe is such an operation ever admissible, for the other toes are so short, and the stumps left by amputation are at once so useless from their shortness, and so detrimental from the manner in which they project upwards and rub against the shoe, that any injury requiring partial amputation of a lesser toe is treated by its complete removal.

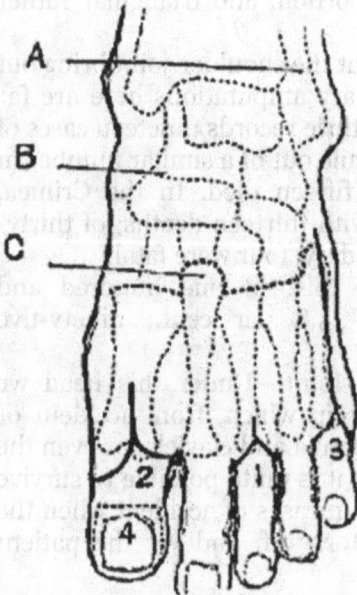

Fig. v.

AMPUTATION OF DISTAL PHALANX OF GREAT TOE.—This is comparatively rarely required now. It used to be thought necessary for the cure of those not uncommon cases of exostosis of the distal phalanx, but it is now found that most of these can be cured by simply clipping off the exostosis. When necessary, however, and when the choice of flaps is possible, the best plan is by a long flap from the plantar surface (Fig. v. 4), as in the similar operation on the thumb; laying the edge of the knife over the dorsal aspect of the joint, cutting through it, and turning the edge of the knife round close to the bone, so as to cut out a large flap from the ball of the toe.

AMPUTATION OF A SINGLE LESSER TOE—second, third, or fourth.—This operation is on exactly the same principle as that

---

[35] Excision of Scapula, p. 33.

described for the corresponding finger; but it must be remembered that the metatarso-phalangeal joint is more deeply situated in the soft parts than is the metacarpo-phalangeal; and thus the commencement of the elliptical incision which is to surround the base of the toe must be proportionally higher up (Fig. v. 1). On the other hand, as it is very important to avoid as much as possible any cicatrix in the sole of the foot, the plantar end of the incision need not be carried to a point exactly opposite the one from which it set out, but it will be sufficient if it reaches the groove between the toe and sole. A little more care may thus be required in dissecting out the head of the first phalanx, but this is quite repaid by the cicatrix in the sole being avoided. Early division of flexor tendons renders disarticulation easy.

AMPUTATION OF THE FIRST AND FIFTH TOES.—The incisions are conducted on the same principle as in the other operations, the operator being careful to preserve as much as possible (Fig. v. 2) of the hard useful pad of the inner and outer sides respectively.

Most surgeons are now agreed that in these toes it is best not to remove the head of the metatarsal bone with the toe. Cutting off the large cartilaginous head obliquely with a pair of bone-pliers may prevent an awkward unseemly projection, but it does diminish the strength of the transverse arch of the foot.

AMPUTATION OF ONE OR MORE TOES WITH THEIR METATARSALS.—It is not necessary to give very particular details regarding such operations, as the surgeon must be guided in the individual cases by the specialties of accident or disease.

One or two guiding principles are important:—

1. Having made up your mind at what point you are to cut the metatarsal, if the amputation be a partial one, or as to the exact position of the joint, if you intend to disarticulate, commence your dorsal incision (Fig. v. 3) at a point fully half an inch higher up than the selected spot, as free access is of the very last importance.

2. Whenever it is possible, cut the bone through its continuity rather than disarticulate. Specially is this important in the case of the metatarsal bone of the great toe, that the insertion of the tendon of the peroneus longus may be saved. If, however, the terminal branch of the dorsalis pedis artery be wounded, it may be necessary to disarticulate the first metatarsal to secure it rather than trust to compression to stop the bleeding.

3. In cutting through the first and fifth metatarsals, remember to apply the bone-pliers obliquely, not transversely, so as to avoid unseemly projection.

4. As far as possible avoid cutting into the sole at all.

The plantar cicatrix is almost a fatal objection to a plan of removing the first and fifth toes and their metatarsals which has much otherwise in rapidity and elegance to recommend it. In the great toe, for example, it is performed as follows:—Seizing the soft parts of the inner edge of the foot in his left hand, the surgeon draws them inwards, transfixes just at the tarso-metatarsal joint, and, keeping as close as possible to the inner edge of the metatarsal bone, cuts the flap as long as to the middle of the first phalanx; then the soft parts of the foot being drawn as far outwards as possible by an assistant, the surgeon enters his knife between the first and second toes, and succeeds in entering his former incision so as to separate the metatarsal bone without removing any skin. All that remains is to open the tarso-metatarsal joint. It is a very neat-looking operation, leaves a very good covering for the parts, and is performed with extreme rapidity. This last is not so much required in these days of anæsthetics, and the cicatrix in the sole is a very formidable objection to it.

The simplest and shortest rule that can be given for the amputation of a toe, with the part or whole of its metatarsal, is to make one dorsal incision, commencing about a quarter of an inch above the spot at which you intend to divide the bone or to disarticulate, extending downwards in a straight line to the metatarso-phalangeal articulation, and then bifurcating so as to surround the base of the toe at the normal fold of the skin. The soft parts are then to be cleared from the metatarso-phalangeal joint, and the toe still being retained on the metatarsal bone, it should be carefully dissected up, avoiding any pricking of the soft parts below, till the joint is reached, or the spot at which the bone-pliers are to be applied is fully cleared.

AMPUTATION OF THE ANTERIOR PORTION OF THE FOOT AT THE TARSO-METATARSAL JOINT—Hey's Operation.—This operation, which is now comparatively rarely performed, has been invested with a halo of difficulty and complexity which is to a great extent unnecessary.

There is no doubt that the anatomical conformation of the joints involved, especially the manner in which the head of the second metatarsal (Fig. v. C) projects upwards into the tarsus, and is locked between the cuneiform bones, renders disarticulation in the healthy foot rather difficult; but it must be remembered that in cases where for accident we have to deal with previously healthy tissues, it is quite unnecessary to disarticulate, a better result being attained by simply sawing the foot across in the line of the articulation; and again, where we have to operate for disease, the tissues are so matted, and the bones so soft, that complete removal of the metatarsus is much easier than it appears when practising on the dead subject.

Very various plans of incision have been proposed. Mr. Hey's original procedure has not been much improved upon. His short account of it has at once surgical value and historical interest:—

"I made a mark across the upper part of the foot, to point out as exactly as I could the place where the metatarsal bones were joined to those of the tarsus. About half an inch from this mark, nearer the toes,

I made a transverse incision through the integuments and muscles covering the metatarsal bones (Plate IV. figs. 10, 11). From each extremity of this wound I made an incision (along the inner and outer side of the foot) to the toes. I removed all the toes at their junction with the metatarsal bones, and then separated the integuments and muscles forming the sole of the foot from the inferior part of the metatarsal bones, keeping the edge of my scalpel as near the bones as I could, that I might both expedite the operation and preserve as much muscular flesh in the flap as possible. I then separated with the scalpel the four smaller metatarsal bones at their junction with the tarsus, which was easily effected, as the joints lie in a straight line across the foot. The projecting part of the first cuneiform bone which supports the great toe I was obliged to divide with a saw. The arteries, which required a ligature, being tied, I applied the flap which had formed the sole of the foot to the integuments which remained on the upper part, and retained them in contact by sutures....

"The patient could walk with firmness and ease; she was in no danger of hurting the cicatrix by striking the place where the toes had been against any hard substance, for this part was covered with the strong integuments which had before constituted the sole of the foot. The cicatrix was situated upon the upper part of the foot, and had very little breadth, as the divided parts had been kept united after being brought into close contact."[36]

Lisfranc's method has, briefly, the following modifications.— Having fixed the position of the articulations of the first and fifth metatarsals with the tarsus, the operator unites them by a curved incision across the dorsum of the foot, with its convexity downwards. He then divides the dorsal ligaments over the articulations, opens the first from the inside, the fifth, fourth, and third from the outside, he then with a strong narrow-bladed knife divides the interosseous ligaments between the sides and end of the head of the second metatarsal and the cuneiforms, thus completing the disarticulation; bending the fore part of the foot downwards, he then keeps the edge of the knife close to the lower surface of the bones, separating the plantar ligaments, and cutting out a long plantar flap of skin and muscles.

In every case it must be remembered that the upper end of the fifth metatarsal projects far up along the outer edge of the foot. Allowance must be made for this projection in commencing the incision. A rule given by Mr. Syme to guide the disarticulation of the three outer metatarsals will often be of service; it is this: "Having once entered the joint of the fifth, the knife must be drawn along in a direction of a line drawn towards the distal end of the first metatarsal; for the fourth, the direction must be changed to the middle of the same

---

[36] Hey's Observations, 3d ed. pp. 552, 556.

51

bone; and to open the third it will be necessary to come across the dorsum of the foot as if intending to reach the proximal end."

To avoid the difficulties of disarticulation, Skey recommends cutting off the head of the second metatarsal with a pair of pliers. Baudens, Guérin, and others approve of sawing all the bones across in the line desired.

Most surgeons are now agreed that in this operation it is better to make both flaps by cutting from without, in preference to transfixion of the plantar one from within. In cases where, from injury and disease, the plantar flap is deficient in size, it may be necessary to make the dorsal flap longer. However, the long plantar is preferable both from its superior hardness, and also because from its length it permits the cicatrix to be well on the dorsum of the foot, and therefore less likely to be injured by the pressure of the boot in front.

AMPUTATIONS THROUGH THE TARSUS.—Various plans of amputating through the tarsus have been devised and described at great length. The most important of these is the operation of removal of the anterior portion of the foot, at the joints between the astragalus and scaphoid, and os calcis and cuboid, well known to the profession by the name of its first describer, Chopart.

It has been so completely superseded by the infinitely preferable amputation at the ankle-joint of Mr. Syme, as rarely, if ever, to be practised in this country. Indeed, amputation at the ankle-joint may be said to have taken the place of all these amputations through the tarsus; for though cases are occasionally met with in which the limitation of the disease or injury may render Chopart's possible, and though at first sight it appears to have an advantage in removing less of the body, still the following objections are nearly fatal to its chance of being selected:—1. In cases of injury, through leaving a long stump, and, at first sight, a useful one, experience shows that the tendo Achillis sooner or later (being unopposed by the extensors of the toes) draws up the heel so as to make the end of the stump point, and the cicatrix press on the ground, rendering it unable to bear any weight. 2. In cases of removal for disease of the tarsus, the bones left behind, though apparently sound at the time, are almost sure to become eventually diseased.

As it has an historical interest, and as this operation (defective as it is) had been the means of saving many legs prior to the invention of amputation at the ankle-joint, a brief description may be appended:—

Chopart's own manner of operation was briefly somewhat as follows:—

The tourniquet having been applied, the surgeon is to make a transverse incision through the skin which covers the instep, two inches from the ankle-joint. He is to divide the skin, and the extensor tendons, and the muscles in that situation, so as to expose the convexity of the tarsus. He is next to make on each side a small

52

longitudinal incision, which is to begin below and a little in front of the malleolus, and is to end at one of the extremities of the first incision. After having formed in this way a flap of integuments, he is to let it be drawn upwards by the assistant who holds the leg. There is no occasion to dissect and reflect the flap, for the cellular substance connecting the skin with the subjacent aponeurosis is so loose, that it can easily be drawn up above the place where the joint of the calcaneum with the cuboides and that between the astragalus and scaphoides ought to be opened. The surgeon will penetrate the last the most easily, particularly by taking for his guide the eminence which indicates the attachment of the tibialis anticus muscle to the inside of the os naviculare. The joint of the os cuboides and os calcis lies pretty nearly in the same transverse line, but rather obliquely forwards. The ligaments having been cut, the foot falls back. The bistoury is then to be put down, and the straight knife used, with which a flap of the soft parts is to be formed under the tarsus and metatarsus, long enough to admit of being applied to the naked bones, so as entirely to cover them. It is to be maintained in position with three or four straps of adhesive plaster, etc.[37]

Chopart's amputation, after an interval of comparative neglect, was introduced into this country by Mr. Syme in 1829. His method of performance is simpler and easier than Chopart's. He thus describes it:—"The blade of the knife employed should be about six inches long, and half an inch broad, sharp at the point and blunt on the back. The tourniquet ought to be applied immediately above the ankle, having compresses placed over the posterior and anterior tibial arteries. The surgeon should measure with his eye the middle distance between the malleolus externus and the head of the metatarsal bone of the little toe, which is the situation of the articulation between the os cuboides and os calcis. Placing his forefinger here, he ought to place his thumb on the other side of the foot directly opposite, which will show him where the os naviculare and astragalus are connected. An incision (Plate II. figs. 4 and 5) somewhat curved, with its convexity forward, is then to be made from one of these points to the other, when, instead of proceeding to disarticulate, the operator should transfix the sole of the foot from side to side at the extremities of the first incision, and carry the knife forwards so as to detach a sufficient flap, which must extend the whole length of the metatarsus to the balls of the toes. The disarticulation may finally be completed with great ease, as the shape of the articular surfaces concerned is very simple, and nearly transverse."[38] Regarding the method of disarticulating at the astragalo-calcaneal joint, and removing all the foot except the astragalus, no detail need be given. Malgaigne advises an internal flap, thus sacrificing the valuable pad of

---

[37] Roux's Parallel between English and French Surgery. Translation abridged from Cooper's Surgical Dictionary, p. 106.
[38] Syme's Principles, 4th edit. p. 145.

the heel. Roux, Verneuil, and others endeavour to save the pad. This operation, however, has now fallen almost completely into disuse.

Subastragaloid Amputation has been highly recommended. In it the flap is made as in Syme's, then anterior bones removed as in Chopart's, and os calcis grasped by lion forceps and twisted off, its attachment and the insertion of tendo Achillis being cautiously avoided. If flaps are scanty, head of astragulus may be cut off with a small saw.—Hancock and Ashurst.

TRIPIER'S AMPUTATION[39] is a modification of above, the skin incisions being made as in Chopart's amputation, and then the calcaneum is sawn through on a level with the sustentaculum tali on a plane at right angles to the axis of the leg.

AMPUTATION AT THE ANKLE-JOINT, OR SYME'S AMPUTATION.—This operation is one of much interest and great practical importance. In our cold variable climate caries of the bones of the tarsus, and strumous disease of the ankle-joint, are very common and very intractable maladies, and for both of these, when far advanced, Syme's amputation is the only justifiable procedure. When properly done, according to the exact plan of its proposer, it removes the whole of the diseased parts and not an inch more, is an operation of very slight danger to life, and results almost invariably in a thoroughly useful comfortable stump. Much of its success depends on the manner in which it is performed, and as many surgical manuals are not sufficiently full, some positively in error regarding this point, and as very many modifications have been devised diminishing in value and applicability very much in proportion as they diverge from the original description, I think it advisable to describe the operation minutely, and point out in detail the parts of it which seem absolutely essential to success.

Operation.—The foot being held at a right angle to the leg, the point of a straight bistoury, with a pretty strong blade, should be entered just below the centre of the external malleolus (Plate IV. figs. 12, 13), (1.) and then carried right across the integuments of the sole, in a straight line (or in the case of a prominent heel, slightly backwards), (2.) to a point at the same level on the opposite side. (3.) This incision should reach boldly through all the tissues down to the bone. Holding the heel in the fingers of his left hand, the operator then inserts his left thumb-nail into the incision, and pushes the flap downwards, as with the knife kept close to the bone, and cutting on it, he frees the flap from its attachments. The thumb-nail guards the knife from in any way scoring the flap. (4.) This process is continued till the tuberosity of the os calcis is fairly turned, and the tendo Achillis nearly reached. Shifting his left hand he then extends the foot, and joins the extremities of the first incision by a transverse one right across the instep. (5.) Thus he

---

[39] International Encyclopædia, vol. 1. p. 655.

54

opens the joint between the astragalus and tibia, (6.) divides the lateral ligaments, disarticulates, and still keeping close to the bone, removes the foot by the division of the tendo Achillis.

The lower ends of the tibia and fibula are then to be isolated from the soft parts, and a thin slice, including both malleoli, to be removed. If the disease of the joint has affected the lower end of the bone, slice after slice may be removed, till a healthy surface of cancellated texture is obtained. The vessels are then secured.

Dressing of the Stump.—From its peculiar shape and position, the escape of any blood into the stump is much to be deprecated, for as it cannot easily get out, on the one hand it gives pain, and may cause sloughing from its pressure, and on the other it is sure eventually to cause suppuration, and delay union. To avoid such results care must be taken to secure every vessel that can be seen; if there is any general oozing it is best merely to pass the sutures through the edges of the flaps, but not bring them together, thus leaving the stump open for some hours; then apply cold, and when the surfaces are fairly glazed over, remove any clots and bring the flaps together.[40]

Another plan introduced by Mr. Syme was to make a longitudinal slit in the flap, through which all the ligatures are to be drawn; these give a dependent drain to any pus that may be formed, and by their presence greatly expedite the healing of the wound. Again, in cases where from the amount of disease existing before the operation, and the gelatinous thickening of the flap and neighbouring parts, much suppuration may be looked for, probably it will be found best to keep the flaps quite apart for some days, by stuffing the wound with lint, and aiming only at secondary union by granulations.

A drainage tube passed through the breadth of the flap, and brought out at the angles, and retained for a few days, will do admirably.

Notes.—(1.) If commenced further forward, as in Pirogoff's modification, it will be found difficult to turn the corner of the heel; if further back, the nutrition of the flap is endangered.

(2.) This is very important. In several well-known text-books, even in the last edition of Gross's Surgery, the incision is figured passing obliquely forwards. This is a fatal error, for besides making a flap far too long, it forces the operator to cut fairly into the hollow of the sole, quite off the prominence of the os calcis, and he finds that it is utterly impossible to free his flap without using great force, and inevitably scoring it in all directions. Sloughing is almost inevitably the result.

(3.) The incision is to stop at least half-an-inch below the internal malleolus. Most surgical manuals, even when they profess to describe Mr. Syme's own method of operating, say that

---

[40] Observations in Clin. Surgery, p. 48.

the incision should extend from malleolus to malleolus. If this is done, the flap becomes unsymmetrical, too long, and also the posterior tibial artery, on which much of the vascular supply of the flap depends, is cut. When the incision is properly made, the vessel is not cut till after its division into the plantar arteries.

(4.) Scoring the flap. Some may ask, Why do you object to a little scoring, the tissues are thick enough, and besides, don't you advise a slit in the flap yourself? Yes. One look at an injected preparation will show that the vessels supplying this thick flap come to it from its inner surface, and are inevitably cut across in any scoring of it, and also, that scoring cuts across the vessels, and must divide dozens of them; the slit we make is parallel with their course, and may not divide one.

(5.) Across the instep. Some authors recommend a semilunar anterior flap; this is quite unnecessary, increases bagging and delays union. It can be required only in cases where the heel flap has been destroyed or lessened by disease, or by operators in whose hands the heel flaps occasionally slough.

(6.) It is not impossible that a careless operator may (by cutting a little too low) miss the joint and get into the hollow of the neck of the astragalus, where he may cut away for a long time without making much progress.

Advantages.—1. It is wonderfully free of danger to life. It is very hard to obtain exact statistical information, but my experience is that the mortality is certainly not more than about 10 per cent., a very remarkable result when compared with that of amputations through the leg, the operation which used to be required for those cases which now require only amputation at the ankle-joint.

In the Statistical Report by the Surgeon-General of the United States, 9705 cases of amputation resulted in death, the proportions being as follows:—

Amputation of hip,	85	er cent. died.
" thigh,	64	
" knee,	55	
" leg,	26	
Amputation of ankle-joint,	13	er cent. died.
" shoulder,	39	
" arm,	21	
" fore-arm,	16	

2. It is the most perfect stump that can be made, in fact the only one in the lower extremity which can bear pressure enough to support

the weight of the body; all the others require the weight to be distributed over the general surface of the limb by means of apparatus. A good ankle-joint stump can bear the whole weight of the body, as when the patient hops on it without any artificial aid, or without even the interposition of a stocking between the stump and a stone floor. More than this, I have seen a patient who had both his feet amputated at the ankle-joint run without shoes or stockings on the stone passages, without even the aid of a stick, and with very great swiftness.

The reason of this may be found in the nature of the flap itself, originally intended to bear the weight of the body, there being no cicatrix at the part on which pressure is borne. I have noticed that perfection in walking on an ankle-joint stump has a certain relation to the freedom of movement which the pad has over the face of the bone. This ought to be pretty considerable. It is explained by the new attachments formed by the tendons, and is under the control of the patient, being elicited when he is told to move his toes.

It has been objected to this operation that the flap is apt to slough. When improperly performed, as when the flap is scored transversely in its separation, and especially when the flap is cut too long (as has been already noticed), this may occur; but that there is nothing whatever in the position or condition of the flap itself that at all necessitates its sloughing, is thoroughly proved by the following remarkable case, given by Mr. Syme in his volume of Observations in Clinical Surgery. I quote it entire:—

"P.C., aged thirty-three, was admitted into the hospital on the 25th July 1860, in the following state:—He had been treated in the Manchester Infirmary for popliteal aneurism by pressure, so decidedly applied that it had caused an ulcer, of which the cicatrix remained; but without producing the effect desired. The femoral artery was then tied with success, in so far as the aneurism was concerned, but with the unpleasant sequel, some months afterwards, of mortification in the foot, which was thrown off, with the exception of the astragalus and os calcis with their integuments, a large raw surface being presented in front where the bone was bare. Although the patient was extremely weak, and the parts concerned might be supposed more than usually disposed to slough, I did not hesitate to perform the operation, with the speedy result of a most excellent stump and complete restoration to health."—Pp. 49, 50.

The modifications of Mr. Syme's original operation have been very various. It will be unnecessary even to name them all. One or two may require notice. Retaining Mr. Syme's incisions in their integrity, some operators prefer not to disarticulate the foot, but remove it by sawing through the tibia and fibula at once, while still in connection with the foot. That most excellent surgeon and first-rate operator, Dr. Johnston of Montrose, used to prefer this method.

In cases where the pad of the heel has been destroyed by disease or accident, so as to be partially or entirely unavailable for the flap, the late Dr. Richard Mackenzie[41] practised the following operation by internal flap:—With the foot and ankle projecting from the table with their internal aspect upwards, he entered the point of the knife (Plate I. fig. 14) in the mesial line of the posterior aspect of the ankle, on a level with the articulation, carried it down obliquely across the tendo Achillis towards the external border of the plantar aspect of the heel, along which it is continued in a semilunar direction. The incision is then curved across the sole of the foot, and terminates on the inner side of the tendon of the tibialis anticus, about an inch in front of the inner malleolus. The second incision (Plate III. fig. 4) is carried across the outer aspect of the ankle in a semilunar direction, between the extremities of the first incisions, the convexity of the incision downwards, and passing half an inch below the external malleolus.

Precisely the same principle might supply the flap from the outer side in cases where the internal flap as well as the heel was deficient, but probably the nutrition of the external flap would be more doubtful. Neither the one nor the other is nearly so good as the true heel flap, and they are both only very poor substitutes for it when it cannot be had.

The modification devised by Dr. Handyside does not seem to have any advantages over the original operation, and has not been adopted.

The modification invented by Professor Pirogoff involves a much more important principle than any of the preceding. Instead of dissecting the flap from the posterior projecting portion of the os calcis, and removing the tarsus entire, he sawed off the posterior portion of the os calcis obliquely, leaving it in contact with the pad of skin, which is retained. Immediately after making the cut which defines the posterior flap and divides the tissues down to the bone, he opens the joint in front, disarticulates, and then putting on a narrow saw immediately behind the astragalus and over the sustentaculum tali, he saws the os calcis obliquely downwards and forwards till he reaches the first incision; then removes the ends of the tibia and fibula and brings up the slice of os calcis into contact with them.

Advantages.—It is easy of performance, saving the dissection from the heel, which some find so hard. It leaves a longer limb. It is said to bear pressure better, and there is certainly not so much chance of bagging of pus, and the mortality is exceedingly small, Hancock's collected cases giving only 8.6 per cent.; in cases of injury it is quite a warrantable operation.

Disadvantages.—It is contrary to sound principle in cases of disease, for it wilfully leaves a portion of the tarsus, in which disease is almost certain to return. It leaves too long a limb, for it is found that

---

[41] Monthly Journal of Medical Science for 1849, vol. ix. p. 951.

the shortening in Mr Syme's method is just sufficient to admit of a properly constructed spring being placed in the boot to make up for the loss of the elastic arch of the foot. It brings the firm pad of the heel too much forward, thus tending to lean the weight of the body on the softer tissues behind the heel. It takes much longer to unite and consolidate.

The author has now, in a large number of cases of Syme's amputation for disease, found advantage in leaving the periosteum in the heel flap, i.e. he cuts fairly into the os calcis when dividing the skin of heel, and then using a periosteum scraper instead of the knife, it is quite easy to remove the whole of the periosteum from the bone; this results in a large and more rounded pad of great strength and thickness.

In cases where from disease or injury it is impossible to obtain either a heel flap or a substitute lateral one, the question is, Where should amputation be performed?

It was for a long time the opinion of nearly all the best surgeons, and still is the opinion of many, that amputation of the leg should be performed at what was known as the "seat of election," just below the knee, even in cases where abundance of soft parts could be obtained for an amputation much lower down. The rule in surgery, to save as much of the body as possible in every amputation, was in the leg believed to be set aside by objections which militated strongly against all the other operations in the leg except the one performed just below the knee. Very briefly, these were somewhat as follows:—1. Just above the ankle you have large bones with nothing to cover them except skin and tendons. 2. Higher up in the calf you have plenty of muscle, but it is all on one side, and that the wrong one; it is very heavy, very difficult to dress and keep in position, and then when you have succeeded with it, the muscle wastes away and the stump is flabby. 3. And chiefly, as in all the amputations of the leg, the cicatrices are so much in the way, and the bones are so ill covered, that the patient can never rest his leg on the stump itself, but has either to rest his weight on his patella impinging on the top of a bottle-shaped leg, or just to stick out his stump behind him and kneel on the top of his wooden leg; therefore it is no use to have a stump longer than a few inches; in fact, the longer the stump is the more it is in the way. And more than this, many of the stumps made near the ankle, or through the calf, are not only useless, but positively painful. The skin becomes attached to the bones, the cicatrix never properly firms at all, the patient can hardly bear the pressure of a stocking, far less can he make use of the limb. For these reasons, secondary amputations below the knee are of very common occurrence.

Now, this idea has been much modified, and a few isolated cases in the past, and series of cases considerably more numerous in the present day, show that under certain conditions, and as a result of certain precautions in their performance, such operations are both warrantable and successful.

In the past, as we find in an erudite note in South's Chelius, Dionis, White, and Bromfield had each of them many successful cases of amputation just above the ankle, successful in so far that artificial limbs could be used which preserved the motion of the knee, and gave the patient much more command of the limb than is possible with the short stump below the knee.

A still more important point to be remembered is, that amputation just above the ankle is a much less fatal amputation than that just below the knee (Lister in Holmes's Surgery, 3d ed. vol. iii. p. 716; Gross, 6th ed. vol. ii. p. 1113; Ben. Bell, 6th edit. vol. vii. p. 312).

There is little doubt, however, that the principle so much in vogue in the present day, of one long anterior or posterior flap, instead of two equal flaps, or of circular amputations, has done very much to make amputations at the ankle or through the calf justifiable and useful in bearing the weight of the body.

AMPUTATION JUST ABOVE THE ANKLE.—Cases admitting of this operation must always be rare, for disease of the tarsus or ankle-joint hardly ever goes so far as to contra-indicate the performance of Mr. Syme's greatly preferable operation; and an accident which would require this operation from injury to the ankle would in most cases require an amputation a good deal higher up from the splintering of the tibia so apt to occur.

In a suitable case the plan of the operation should be as follows:—A long anterior flap slightly rounded at the end should be cut (Plate I. figs. 15, 16)—from the outside, not by transfixion,—and the anterior muscles dissected up along with it. It should be long enough to fall down over the face of the bones at the point of section, and easily cover the point of the posterior flap, which is to be made by cutting through all the tissues with one bold transverse stroke of the knife. This operation, which is the plan of Mr. Teale of Leeds very slightly modified, is equally applicable at any point of the leg, with this difference only, that the length of the anterior flap must always be carefully proportioned to the mass of the muscular flap behind it has to cover in.

This operation provides a skin covering, without any danger of the cicatrix being pressed on or becoming adherent.

The author has within the last few years operated nine times in this manner, in cases of accident in which the heel flaps had been completely destroyed; and seen a tenth case in which Mr. Syme did so. All ten cases recovered completely and rapidly, and walked on useful limbs, with the free movement of the knee-joint.

Where from injury in a muscular patient a long anterior flap cannot be had, recourse should be had at once to the operation at the seat of election, rather than run the risk of pressure on the cicatrix by using a double flap operation, or trust that broken reed, the long posterior flap from the great muscles of the calf.

In June 1865, Mr. Henry Lee described a method of operating which he hoped would unite the benefits of Mr. Teale's method to the ease of performance of the old flap from the calf. I append a short account of his method. From its position, however, it has the great disadvantage of retaining the discharges, and by its weight straining the stitches and weighing down the cicatrix:—

LEE'S AMPUTATION *of the Leg by a long rectangular flap from the Calf.*—The operation described was performed according to Mr. Teale's method, as far as the external incisions were concerned, but the long flap was made from the back instead of from the front of the limb (Plate IV. figs. 14, 15). Two parallel incisions were made along the sides of the leg, these were met by a third transverse incision behind, which joined the lower extremities of the first two. These incisions, which formed the three sides of the square, extended through the skin and cellular tissue only. A fourth incision was made transversely through the skin in front of the leg so as to form a flap in this situation, one-fourth only of the length of the posterior flap. When the skin had somewhat retracted by its natural elasticity, an incision was made through the parts situated in front of the bones, which were reflected upwards to a level with the upper extremities of the first longitudinal incisions. The deeper structures at the back of the leg were then freely divided in the situation of the lower transverse incision. The conjoined gastrocnemius and soleus muscles were separated from the subjacent parts, and reflected as high as the anterior flap. The deeper layer of muscles, together with the large vessels and nerves, were divided as high as the incision would permit, and the bones sawn through in the usual way. The flaps were then adjusted in the manner recommended by Mr. Teale.[42]

The patients were able to bear the weight of the body on the end of the stump.

In cases of chronic disease, where the muscles are atrophied and condensed, the following posterior flap method may be used with advantage. It is approved of by Mr. Spence. An incision is made across the front of the leg from the posterior edge of the fibula to the posterior edge of the tibia, or vice versâ, according to the limb. The limb is then transfixed behind the bones from the same points, and a long and gently rounded posterior flap cut. The bones are then cleaned, and cut through at a little higher level.

AMPUTATION IMMEDIATELY BELOW THE KNEE *at the "true seat of election."*—The principles on which this operation is founded are—1. That a muscular flap is not necessary, skin being perfectly sufficient; 2. That as the muscles retract they must be cut at a lower

---

[42] Med. Times and Gazette, June 3, 1865.

level than the bones, and as they retract unequally from their varying length, the cuts must be made with due reference to that inequality; 3. That no more of the tibia need be retained than what is just sufficient to retain the attachment of the ligamentum patellæ, and to insure its vitality; 4. That the head of the fibula must be retained in every case, as in a certain proportion the tibio-fibular articulation communicates with the knee-joint.

Operation.—Two equal semilunar flaps of skin must be cut— from the outside, not by transfixion,—one anterior and external, the other posterior and internal, their extremities meeting at points about two inches below the tuberosity of the tibia on either side (Plate I. figs. 17, 18). These must be reflected up, and with them a further extent of skin, embracing the whole circumference of the limb, must be dissected up (as if pulling off the fingers of a glove), so as to expose the bone one inch below the tuberosity. The anterior muscles being very close to their origin, and consequently being able to retract very slightly, must be cut as high as exposed, and the posterior ones about the middle of their exposed surface.

The bones must then be sawn as high as exposed, with the following precautions:—1. In order to prevent splintering of the fibula, endeavour to saw it along with the tibia, so as to finish it first; 2. To prevent projection of a sharp prominence of the edge of the tibia, enter the saw obliquely a little higher up than where you intend to divide the bone, then withdraw it, and enter the saw again at right angles to the bone, and a line or two lower down. Some surgeons prefer to make this section afterwards with a finer saw or the bone-pliers.

This operation is very frequently required to remedy painful and unhealed stumps, the result of amputations lower down, specially those in which the long posterior flap from the muscles of the calf has been used. In the above amputation the patient will not be able to rest the weight of his body on the face of the stump, but by putting the limb into a well-padded case with soft rounded edges, the weight might be borne partly on the sides of the stump, and partly on the lower edge of the patella; and the patient will be able to walk with great comfort, preserving the use of his knee-joint.

AMPUTATION AT THE KNEE-JOINT.—This "relic of ancient surgery," as Mr. Skey calls it, has been revived only of late years, and seems in certain cases to be a justifiable and successful operation.

Practised by Fabricius Hildanus and Guillemeau in the sixteenth and seventeenth centuries, it had fallen into disuse till revived by Hoin, Velpeau, and Baudens, on the Continent, Professor Nathan Smith in America, and Mr. Lane in London.

It is not possible that this operation can be at all frequent, since the cases in which it is applicable are comparatively rare; for, to be successful, the following conditions are essential:—1. That there be abundant skin in front of the knee-joint to make a long anterior flap; 2.

That the patella and articular surface of the femur are healthy. These conditions at once exclude nearly every case of disease or accident. If the joint is diseased some amputation through the thigh must be attempted; if injured, and the front of the knee is safe, it may very likely be possible to amputate below the knee. Hence this operation may be useful in cases where, for malignant disease, the whole tibia requires removal, and yet the knee-joint is sound, or for gunshot injuries, in which the tibia is splintered but the soft tissues comparatively uninjured.

Operation.—A long anterior flap should be cut with a semilunar end (Plate II. figs. 6, 7), extending as far as the insertion of the ligamentum patellæ. This flap, including the patella, should be thrown up, the joint cut into, and a short posterior flap made by transfixion.

It is important to retain the patella, if possible, as it fills up the hollow between the condyles; it sometimes becomes anchylosed, but in other cases it remains freely mobile, and adds to the value of the stump.

Professor Pancoast has practised an amputation at the knee-joint by three flaps, performed entirely by the scalpel, which, he says, results in a good stump. One flap, the anterior one, is longest and semilunar in shape, its convexity passing three inches below the tuberosity of the tibia; the other two are much smaller, and postero-lateral.[43]

Advantages.—The bone is not cut into at all, there is a free drain for matter, no tendency to retraction of the flaps, and the weight of the body is borne on skin previously habituated to pressure.

The statistics seem to be favourable: out of 55 cases, Continental, American, and English, 21 died, a mortality of 38 per cent., while in a table of 1055 cases of amputation of the thigh, 464 died, being a mortality of 44 per cent. In some of the American cases the articulating extremity of the femur seems to have been removed, as in the following operation:—

AMPUTATION THROUGH THE CONDYLES OF THE FEMUR.—In the London and Edinburgh Journal of Medical Science for 1845, Mr. Syme advocated a method of amputation through the condyles of the femur as specially suitable in case of diseased knee-joint. Amputation at this spot has certain advantages:—1. The shaft of the bone being untouched, there is no injury of the medullary cavity, and hence no fear of inflammation of its lining membrane. 2. There is less risk of exfoliation, the cancellated texture of the epiphysis not being liable to it. 3. Being close to the joint, the muscles are cut through where they are tendinous, thus very much diminishing the risk of retraction and consequent protrusion of the bone. 4. A large broad surface of bone is left to bear the weight of the body, and one which,

---

43 Operative Surgery, p. 170.

63

like the ankle-joint stump, will round off and afford a comfortable pad over which the skin of the flap will freely play.

One objection used to be urged against this mode of operating, the fear lest the thickened, brawny, and often ulcerated textures in the neighbourhood of a diseased knee-joint, would not make a good covering. This, however, is no longer a bugbear, as we see in cases of resection, where the diseased joint alone is taken away, how very soon all swelling and disease departs, once its cause is removed.

Mr. Syme's original operation was briefly as follows:—With an ordinary amputating-knife make a lunated incision (Plate I. fig. 19) from one condyle to the other, across the front of the joint, on a level with the middle of the patella, divide the tissues down to the bones, and then draw the flap upwards, then cut the quadriceps extensor immediately above the patella. The point of the blade should then be pushed in at one end of the wound, thrust behind the femur, and made to appear at the other end; it should then be carried downwards (Plate III. fig. 5), so as to make a flap from the calf of the leg, about six or eight inches in length, in proportion to the thickness of the limb; the flap should then be slightly retracted, and the knife carried round the bone a little above the condyles to clear a way for the saw, which should be applied so as to leave the section as horizontal as possible.

This method is now hardly ever used, as the following seems a much better one:—

GRITTI'S[44] AMPUTATION.—In this two flaps are formed—an anterior long one rectangular and a posterior short one. The condyles of the femur are divided through their base, and the lower surface of patella is removed by a small saw, and then the surfaces of bone approximated.

STOKES'S[45] MODIFICATION OF GRITTI'S AMPUTATION.—In this "supracondyloid" amputation, the femur is sawn just above the condyles, without going into the medullary canal. The anterior flap is oval, twice as long as posterior, and the patella is brought up after denudation against end of femur.

CARDEN'S AMPUTATION AT THE CONDYLES OF THE FEMUR.[46]—The operation consists in reflecting a rounded or semi-oval flap of skin and fat from the front of the knee-joint, dividing everything else straight down to the bone, and sawing the bone slightly above the plane of the muscles, thus forming a flat-faced stump, with a bonnet of integument to fall over it.

The operator standing on the right side of the limb, seizes it between his left forefinger and thumb at the spot selected for the base of the flap, and enters (Plate II. fig. 8) the point of the knife close to his

---

44 Annali Universali de Medicina, Milano, 1857.

45 Med. Chir. Transactions of London, vol. liii., p. 175.

46 Carden's (of Worcester) Pamphlet, pp. 5, 6; and British Medical Journal, 1864.

finger, bringing it round through skin and fat below the patella to the spot pressed by his thumb; then turning the edge downwards at a right angle with the line of the limb, he passes it through to the spot where it first entered, cutting outwards through everything behind the bone (Plate IV. fig. 16). The flap is then reflected, and the remainder of the soft parts divided straight down to the bone; the muscles are then slightly cleared upwards, and I saw it applied.

I have ventured to make a slight change in the method of performing this most excellent operation, for having found the posterior flap, as cut in the method above described, rather scanty in the earlier cases in which I have had occasion to perform it, after dissecting back the anterior flap and cutting into the knee-joint, I shape a slightly convex posterior flap of skin only, at least one and a half inches in length in adult, and allow it to retract before dividing the muscles by a circular cut to the bone, and have had every reason to be satisfied with the change.

Amputation of the Thigh.—Amputation of the thigh has been the favourite battle-ground where flap and circular, antero-posterior and lateral, long and short flaps, double, triple, and conical incisions, have striven with each other; so were I to attempt to describe one quarter of the various methods employed, I should need to rewrite the history of Amputation.

It will suffice merely to describe the best modes of amputating the thigh through its lower, middle, and upper thirds respectively, and at the hip-joint.

In one word, it may be stated that, with the exception of those amputations performed through the lower third of the bone, the flap method is to be preferred, and the flaps should in almost every case be made by transfixion.

In the lower third, however, the flap method, though exceedingly easy, and capable of very rapid performance, has certain defects; the chief of these being the tendency which the muscular flaps (the necessary result of transfixion) have to cause undue retraction, and hence protrusion of the bone. This is seen specially in the hamstrings, which from the great distance of their origin, and the purely longitudinal direction of their fibres, retract to a very great extent, much more than the anterior muscles can do from the pennate direction of their fibres, and the manner in which they are mutually bound down to each other and to the bone.

Even in this one position, the lower third of the thigh, the methods that may be needed are various, and require separate notice;— for operations here are extremely frequent from the frequency of strumous disease of the knee-joint in our variable climate, and from the fact that compound fractures or dislocations of the knee-joint so very often necessitate amputation.

In cases where the skin over the patella is uninjured and

available, the operation by long anterior flap (either by Teale's method, or by Mr. Spence's modification of it, which curiously is almost exactly similar to the amputation of Benjamin Bell by a single flap) is suitable enough. But, I believe, preferable to either of these is the operation of Mr. Carden, already described. In cases where the knee-joint is injured, and the skin over the patella unavailable, and yet where it is not necessary to go higher up the limb, the modified circular amputation of Mr. Syme will be found very suitable.

As it is in this lower third of the thigh that a very large proportion of the cases requiring a long anterior flap is to be found, it affords the best opportunity for comparing in their detail the three almost similar plans of B. Bell, Teale, and Spence—after which Mr. Syme's modified circular may be described.

BENJAMIN BELL'S FLAP OPERATION ABOVE THE KNEE (reported in his own words, slightly abbreviated).—"When this operation is to be performed above the knee, it may be done either with one or two flaps, but it will commonly succeed best with one. The flap answers best on the fore part of the thigh, for here there is a sufficiency of the parts for covering the bones, and the matter passes more freely off than when the flap is formed behind.... The extreme point of the flap should reach to the end of the limb, unless the teguments are in any part diseased, in which case it must terminate where the disease begins, and its base should be where the bone is to be sawn. This will determine the length of the flap, and we should be directed with respect to the breadth of it by the circumference of the limb, for the diameter of a circle being somewhat less than a third of its circumference, although a limb may not be exactly circular, yet by attention to this we may ascertain with sufficient exactness the size of a flap for covering a stump (Plate IV. fig. 17). Thus a flap of four inches and a quarter in length will reach completely across a stump whose circumference is twelve inches; but as some allowance must be made for the quantity of skin and muscles that may be saved on the opposite side of the limb, by cutting them in the manner I have directed, and drawing them up before sawing the bone, and as it is a point of importance to leave the limb as long as possible, instead of four inches and a quarter, a limb of this size, when the first incision is managed in this manner, will not require a flap longer than three inches and a quarter, and so in proportion, according to the size of the limb. The flap at its base should be as broad as the breadth of the limb will permit, and should be continued nearly, although not altogether, of the same breadth till within a little of its termination, where it should be rounded off so as to correspond as exactly as may be with the figure of the sore on the back part of the limb. This being marked out, the surgeon, standing on the outside of the limb, should push a straight double-edged knife with a sharp point to the depth of the bone, by entering the point of it at the outside of the base of the intended flap; and carrying

66

the point close to the bone, it must here be pushed through the teguments at the mark on the opposite side. The edge of the knife must now be carried downwards in such a direction as to form the flap, according to the figure marked out; and as it draws toward the end, the edge of it should be somewhat raised from the bone, so as to make the extremity of the flap thinner than the base, by which it will apply with more neatness to the surface of the sore. The flap being supported by an assistant, the teguments and muscles of the other parts of the limb should, by one stroke of the knife, be cut down to the bone, about an inch beneath where the bone is to be sawn; and the muscles being separated to this height from the bone with the point of a knife, the soft parts must all be supported with the leather retractors till the bone is sawn," etc., arteries tied, and dressings applied.[47]

AMPUTATION OF THIGH BY RECTANGULAR FLAP— (Teale's).—I take the opportunity here of describing fully, and as far as possible in his own words, Mr. Teale's method of amputating, this being the situation where his method is most frequently available. The same principle may be applied to amputations at almost any other part of the body.

After advising the surgeon to mark out the proposed line of incision with ink before the operation, he gives the following directions for fixing the exact size of the flap:—"Supposing the amputation to take place (Plate II. figs. 9, 10) at the lower part of the middle third of the thigh, the circumference of the limb is to be measured at the point where the bone is to be divided.[48] Assuming this to be sixteen inches, the long flap is to have its length and breadth each equal to half the circumference, namely, eight inches. Two longitudinal lines of this extent are then traced on the limb, and are met at their lower points by a transverse line of the same length. The inner longitudinal line should be first traced in ink as near as practicable to the femoral vessels, without including them within the range of the long flap. The outer longitudinal line, which is somewhat posterior, is next marked eight inches distant from the former and parallel to it. These two lines are then joined by a transverse line of the same extent, which falls upon the upper border of the patella, or upon some lower portion of this bone. The short flap is indicated by a transverse line passing behind the thigh, the length of this flap being one-fourth that of the long one; or, assuming the circumference of the limb to be sixteen inches, and the length of the long flap eight inches, the length of the short flap is two inches. The operator begins by making the two lateral incisions of the long flap through the integuments only. The transverse incision of this flap, supposing it to run along the upper edge of the patella, is made by a free sweep of the knife through the skin and tendinous structures

---

[47] B. Bell's Surgery, 6th ed. vol. vii. pp. 336-339.
[48] In diagram the amputation is drawn as if for middle third of thigh.

down to the femur. Should the lower transverse line of the flap fall across the middle or lower part of the patella, the transverse incision can extend through the skin only, which must be dissected up as far as the upper border of the patella, at which place the tendinous structures are to be cut direct to the thigh-bone. The flap is completed by cutting the fleshy structures from below upwards close to the bone. The posterior short flap, containing the large vessels and nerves, is made by one sweep of the knife down to the bone, the soft parts being afterwards separated from the bone close to the periosteum, as far upwards as the intended place of sawing.... In adjusting the flaps, the long one is folded over the end of the bone, and brought, by its transverse line, into union with the short flap, the two corresponding free angles of each being first united by suture. One or two additional stitches complete the transverse line of union. Care is now required in arranging the two lateral lines of union. As the long flap is folded upon itself so as to form a kind of pouch for the end of the bone, it is requisite that it should be held in its folded state by a point of suture on each side. Another stitch on each side secures the lateral line of the short flap to the corresponding part of the long one. A longitudinal line of union thus passes at right angles each end of the transverse line."[49]

Mr. Teale's account of the resulting stumps is too long to quote entire, but in a few words, we find that by retraction of the short posterior flap, the cicatrix is drawn up quite behind and out of the way of the bone, that a soft mass without any large nerves or vessels is the result of the partial atrophy of the long flap, and that the patient is able to bear one-half, two-thirds, or even in some cases the entire weight of his body on the face of the stump. Such a power of support is to be found in no other flap except in Mr. Syme's amputation at the ankle-joint.

SPENCE'S AMPUTATION BY A LONG ANTERIOR FLAP.[50]— The method used by Mr. Spence in amputations just above the knee-joint obtains the advantages of Teale's method, and avoids many of its disadvantages. He makes two flaps. The anterior one, which is to fall loosely over and cover in the posterior segment of the stump, must have a breadth fully equal to one-half of the circumference of the limb, and must be gently rounded at its extremity, so as to adjust itself readily to the curve of the cut margin of the posterior half of the stump. He begins the anterior incision below, or on a level with, the lower margin of the patella, and when the skin is retracted to a little above the patella, cuts down obliquely to the bone, so as to divide the soft parts up to the base of the flap. For the posterior incision, he begins about two fingers'-breadth below the base of the anterior flap, and the assistant retracting the skin, the edge of the knife is carried obliquely

---

[49] Teale, op. cit., pp. 34, 39.
[50] Edin. Med. Journal, for April 1863.

up to the bone (in Alanson's manner) and the posterior soft parts divided, the bone is sawn through—or immediately above—the condyloid portion. Mr. Spence does not advise or practise this method high up. The results are good, for by these means the end of the bone has a thick covering, including muscular fibres, over it, and the cicatrix is not pressed upon in walking. The stump remains full, mobile, and fleshy, as in Mr. Teale's method, without the disadvantage which it has, in requiring the bone to be divided so far above the seat of injury or disease. This is an exceedingly good method of operating in the lower third of the thigh, in muscular patients the very best, and in all cases only equalled in value by Carden's method.

The next is now hardly ever used here, except in cases where the skin over the patella is destroyed.

MODIFIED CIRCULAR AT LOWER THIRD OF THIGH (Syme's).—Two equal semilunar flaps of skin should be cut (Plate I. fig. 20, Plate III. fig. 6), one anterior, the other posterior, their convexities being towards the knee. The skin and subcutaneous cellular tissue should be raised from the fascia, and then retracted to a further distance of at least two inches; the muscles should then be divided right down to the bone, on a level as high as they are exposed in front, and as low as they are exposed behind. This allows for the different amount of retraction at the two sides of the limb, and leaves the muscles cut on a level; the whole mass of muscles should then be drawn well up, and the bone exposed, and sawn through at a level about two inches higher than where it was first exposed by the anterior incision through the muscles.

In very weak thin flabby limbs this process may be simplified by just at once including the muscles in the skin flaps, and carefully exposing the bone higher up. In performing the retraction the assistant should be cautioned not to overdo it, lest he strip the periosteum from the bone higher than is necessary. This is very easy to do in the weak limbs of strumous patients, and may cause exfoliation, and greatly delay cure.

AMPUTATION IN THE MIDDLE THIRD OF THE THIGH.—A very short notice will suffice here. The exact position, shape, and size of the flaps must in every case be modified by the nature of the injury for which the operation is performed, taking the flaps where they can be obtained. As a general rule, a long anterior flap with a short posterior, on the principle described above, should be preferred. In cases where the long anterior cannot be obtained, two equal flaps should be made by transfixion. The flaps should always be antero-posterior, the lateral flaps introduced by Vermale, and indorsed by Chelius and Erichsen, having the great disadvantage of allowing the bone, which is drawn up by the psoas and iliacus, to project at the upper angle.

Supposing the right thigh is to be amputated, the surgeon, standing on the inside of the leg, should raise the skin and muscles of the front of the limb in his left hand, and entering the knife just in front of the vessels, should transfix the limb, the knife passing in front of the bone, and including as nearly as possible an exact half of the limb (Plate IV. fig. 19); having by a sawing motion brought out the knife and cut a flap of the required length, the knife is re-entered at the same place, and passing behind the bone, the point must be brought out at the angle on the other side. Both flaps being then held back by an assistant, the bone is cleared by a circular turn of the knife, and the saw applied, the vessels are found cut high up in the inner angle of the posterior flap.

In muscular patients it is often better to make the incision through the skin first and allow it to retract before transfixing; this is slower and not so brilliant looking, but avoids redundancy of muscle.

AMPUTATION AT THE HIP-JOINT.—This operation, exceedingly dangerous from the amount of the body removed, the great hæmorrhage, and the risk of pyæmia, is of comparatively modern invention. Though the proportion of recoveries is at present to that of deaths about one to two or two and a half, it is still a perfectly justifiable operation in many cases of disease and injury.

Like amputation at the shoulder, amputation at the hip has given rise to very many various methods of performance. Under the heads of single flap, double flap, oval, circular, and mixed flap and circular, at least twenty distinct methods have been put on record, and, including modifications, there are thirty-seven or thirty-eight different surgeons who have each their own plan of operation.

The reason of this fearful complexity in its literature depends on this fact, that this amputation has generally been performed for cases of such severe injury of the limb, that no milder amputation was possible, and thus the flaps had to be taken just where the surgeon could get them best. And this will have to be the guiding principle in most amputations at this joint; the surgeon must just cut his coat according to his cloth—get his flaps where and how he can.

In cases, however, where it is possible to have a choice, and to select the flaps, the following is, I believe, both the best and quickest method:—

This is one of the very few operations in which quickness of performance is a desideratum; the use of anæsthetics has, in most other cases, given time for elaboration of flaps, and careful dissection; here the risk of loss of blood, specially from the posterior flap, renders rapid disarticulation imperative.

Amputation by double flap, anterior the longer.—In hip-joint amputations, besides the ordinary sponge-squeezers, two assistants are necessary, whose duties are exceedingly important.

The first is to check hæmorrhage. Pressing with a firm pad on the external iliac just as it passes the bone, he must be prepared, the instant the anterior flap is cut, to follow the knife and seize flap and artery in his hand, and he is to hold it there till all the vessels in the posterior flap are first tied.

The second has to manage the limb, and on the manner in which he performs his duty much of the success and nearly all the celerity of the operation depend. While the surgeon is transfixing the anterior flap, this assistant is to support the limb in a slightly flexed position, so as to relax the muscles; the instant the flap is cut he is to extend the limb forcibly, and at the same time be careful not to abduct it in the least, but to turn the toes inward so as to bring the great trochanter well forwards on a level with the joint; if this precaution is neglected, the operator in making the posterior flap is almost certain to lock his knife in the hollow between the head of the bone and the great trochanter.

If it is the left side, the operator, standing on the outside of the limb, enters the point of a long straight knife midway between the anterior superior spinous process of the ilium and the great trochanter, and passes it as close to the front of the joint as possible, making the point emerge close to the tuberosity of the ischium (Plate IV. fig. 20-20). With a rapid sawing movement he then cuts a long anterior flap, avoiding any pointing of it, and endeavouring to make the curve equal. The fingers of the assistant must be inserted so as to follow the knife and seize the vessel even before it is divided. The flap being raised out of the way, the surgeon, without changing his knife (as used to be advised), opens the joint, divides the ligaments as they start up on the limb being extended and adducted, the round ligament, and the posterior part of the capsule; and then getting the knife fairly behind both the head of the bone and the trochanter, cuts the posterior flap as rapidly as possible. Instantly on the limb being separated, assistants should be ready with large dry sponges or pads of dry lint to press against the surface of the posterior flap, till the large branches, chiefly of the internal iliac, which are cut in it, are tied one by one.

The lever invented by Mr. Richard Davy, by which the common iliac is compressed from the rectum, has in many cases proved of great service in preventing hæmorrhage, but has dangers of its own in cases of abnormal position of rectum, or even in sudden movements of the patient.

In every case the abdominal tourniquet will be found of great service in checking hæmorrhage, during the operation of amputation at the hip-joint. It consists of an arch of steel fitted with a pad behind, which rests against the vertebral column, and a pad in front playing on a very fine and long screw, through an opening in the arch. When screwed down tightly on the aorta just before the incisions are commenced, it checks hæmorrhage admirably without injuring the viscera. When this is applied, a method of amputation once practised by Mr. Syme, though not so rapid as the double-flap method by transfixion, will be found very easy, and to result in most excellent flaps. He cut an anterior flap in the usual manner by transfixion, then made a straight incision from its outer edge down to about two inches below the great trochanter, thus exposing it fully, and from the lower end of this incision transfixed again, cutting a posterior flap nearly equal in size to the anterior; a few strokes of the knife round the joint finished the disarticulation. The resulting flaps came together with great accuracy, and were not burdened with the great unequal masses of muscles so often noticed in the posterior flaps which are made by cutting from within outwards after disarticulation.

In some cases of amputation where the femur has been badly shattered, it is a good plan to amputate through the upper third of thigh, tie all the vessels, and then, aided by an incision at outer side, dissect out the head of the bone.

Mr. Furneaux Jordan of Birmingham carries out this principle by first dividing the soft parts in circular direction low down the thigh, and then dissecting out the head of the bone from the muscles by a long incision on the outer aspect of the limb.

Note.—In severe cases of smash when both lower limbs have required amputation, the author has derived much assistance from the method of managing the operation detailed below:—

Double Primary Amputation of (both) Thighs from railway smash—Rapid recovery.—G., a healthy-looking man, aged twenty-seven, but looking much older, while driving a horse near Granton, caught his foot on the edge of a rail at a point, fell, and both his legs were run over by several loaded wagons. A special engine was procured, his thighs tightly tied up, and he was sent up to hospital at once.

I was in hospital at the time, so with as little delay as possible he was placed on the operating table, and the necessity for amputation being too evident, I obtained his leave to remove both his legs above the knee; but his pulse was very feeble, and he was intensely nervous, throwing his arms wildly about, panting for breath, and looking very ill, cold, and exhausted.

I determined that by great rapidity he might be got off the table alive, so operated in the following manner:—Fixing the tourniquet firmly near both groins, I first amputated the right leg by Carden's method, and tied the femoral only, wrapped up the stump in a towel wrung out of carbolic solution 1-20, then took off the other limb by Mr. Spence's method,—it had been injured higher than the right, so that I could not save the condyles of the femur,—then tied the femoral there, and fixed it up with another towel; then returning to the first, I tied one or two large branches which spouted, and rolled it up again, then back to the left one, doing the same, and getting the tourniquet off both limbs. On going back to the right the surface was nearly dry and glazed, so, asking Dr. Maclaren, who assisted me, to stitch it up and insert a

72

drainage-tube, I did the same for the left, so rapidly that the patient was in his bed with his limbs dressed and bandaged in 24½ minutes from the time he entered the hospital gate.

The strictest antiseptic precautions were observed, two engines being used to furnish spray. Of course this great rapidity was due to the fact that everything was ready, the assistants all in hospital, admirably disciplined, and steam had been up in the spray engines. Shock was comparatively trivial; his temperature once, and only once, reached 100°. His stumps healed by first intention, and he was in the garden on the seventh day after the operation.

I have now in three cases found the benefit of this mode of dealing with double primary amputation in avoiding shock, lessening the time needed, and greatly diminishing the number of vessels requiring to be tied. In a previous case of double amputation for railway smash at the knees, the patient was almost pulseless, and had he been kept many minutes more on the table would not have left it alive. He also rapidly recovered.

The case is interesting also as showing that, when the assistants know their work, the strictest adherence to antiseptic precautions need not in itself make either the operation or the dressing tedious, though it can easily be made an excuse for much fussing and many delays.[51]

---

[51] Edin. Medical Journal, March 1879.

CHAPTER III

EXCISION OF JOINTS

Historical.—Beyond a passage ascribed to Hippocrates, but of very doubtful authenticity, and slight allusions in the works of Celsus and Paulus Ægineta, the ancients give us no information whatever on this subject.

Hippocrates says,—"Complete resections of bones in the neighbourhood of joints both in the foot, in the hand, in the tibia up to the malleoli, and in the ulna at its junction with the hand, and in many other places, are safe operations, if that fatal syncope does not at once occur, and continued fever does not attack the patient on the fourth day."

Celsus and Ægineta both advise the removal of protruding ends of bone in compound dislocations, but without giving any cases.

From the days of these classic fathers of Surgery, we have hardly an indication of any attention whatever having been paid to their hints till quite within the last hundred years.

The first distinct publication on the subject was by Henry Park of Liverpool, in a letter to Percival Pott in 1783. He proposed the removal of the articulating extremities of diseased elbow and knee-joints to obtain cures. He says he was led to this by its having been the invariable custom, for more than thirty years, at the Liverpool Infirmary, to take off the protruded extremities of bones in cases of compound dislocation.

The chief credit, however, in practically elevating excisions into the catalogue of recognised surgical operations, is owing, British surgeons most cordially own, to two provincial surgeons of France, the Moreaus (father and son) of Bar-sur-Ornain. They took the lead in the most marked manner, having excised the shoulder in 1786, the wrist and elbow in 1794, knee and ankle in 1792, and had followed this up so well that, in 1803, the younger Moreau could boast, "the town has become in some sort the refuge of the unfortunate afflicted with carious joints, after they have tried all the means usually recommended by professional men, or have had recourse to empirical nostrums, or when amputation seemed to them the last resource."

Moreau's papers and cases, which, between 1786 and 1789, he frequently read to the French Academy, were, some violently opposed, others utterly neglected by his compatriots, and many of them lost and buried in the unpublished papers of that body.

And though diseased joints did not decline in frequency, and

74

though injured ones were extremely numerous during these long years of European war, excisions were but rarely performed.

With the exception of the removal of head of humerus after gunshot injury, hardly any British, and but very few French, limbs were saved by excision taking the place of amputation.

The limbs that were saved by Percy by excision of the head of the humerus really owe their recovery and safety to the elder Moreau; for an operation of his, at which he was assisted by that distinguished military surgeon, gave the latter the hint, which he followed so successfully, that by 1795 he had performed it nineteen times, and had indoctrinated Sabatier, Larrey, and others, and elevated it into a recognised operation of military surgery.

So far, however, as the application of the great improvement of the Moreaus to disease went, the French surgeons have little reason to boast, for it is to English surgery, and especially to one Edinburgh surgeon, that this class of operations owes nearly all its improvement in methods and frequency of performance.

For though (as we shall see under the special heads) here and there one or two cases were performed, it was not till the publication of Mr. Syme's monograph on the excision of diseased joints, in 1831, that the importance and value of the discovery were fairly brought before the profession; and the conservative surgery, of which excision as preferred to amputation is the great type, must ever be associated with British surgeons—Syme, Fergusson, Mackenzie, Jones of Jersey, Butcher of Dublin.

On the Continent—Langenbeck, Stromeyer, Heyfelder, Ollier, Esmarch of Kiel, specially in the surgical history of the first Schleswig-Holstein war, have followed up the example set them here.

Before proceeding to describe the operations on the various joints, one or two questions may be briefly asked and answered by way of introduction.

In what cases, or sorts of cases, are excisions suitable?

1. In cases of compound injury or dislocation of a large joint, as used by Filkin, Park, White, and other English surgeons long ago. In hospital practice, or in private, where there is every advantage of rest, food, and appliances, such operations will frequently be found suitable where the joint is alone or chiefly the seat of injury, and where the general health seems fit to bear a prolonged suppuration. But long and sad experience has shown that, as a general rule in military practice, with the difficulties of transport, the generally bad sanitary state of the hospitals, and the want often of adequate dressings and attention, excisions are much more fatal than amputations, and, except in elbow and shoulder (q.v.), should be as a general rule avoided.

2. Excision for deformity (generally speaking for bony anchylosis) will require for decision the consideration of many points, i.e. the joint affected, the nature of the disease or injury which has

caused the anchylosis: and in each case—(1.) the state of health of the patient; and (2.) his occupation, and the consequent position of limb which would suit him best. As a general rule, I believe, experience will prove that such operations on the lower extremity are almost absolutely inadmissible, except under very special urgency on the part of the patient, and a very high condition of health—while in the upper, the elbow-joint is the only one which you will ever be likely to be asked to remedy, or should comply with the request if asked; as the shoulder, even if anchylosed, will (1.) from its own weight generally become so in the most favourable position; and (2.) from the extreme mobility which the scapula can acquire, its anchylosis will not be so much felt.

The elbow, however, from the frequency of fractures of the condyles of the humerus obliquely into the joint, and from the manner in which these are so often neither recognised nor properly treated, very often becomes anchylosed in the most awkward possible position, i.e. nearly straight; and operations undertaken for such deformities are in general both quite safe and very satisfactory. Mr. Syme had one case (resulting from a fall, causing a double fracture), in which both arms were thus firmly anchylosed in such a position that the sufferer could absolutely perform none of the commonest duties of life without assistance. Excision of both joints cured him.

The author excised with success for disease the elbow-joint of a patient whose other arm had required the same operation.

The occupation of the patient must always be taken into consideration when settling the position of an anchylosis, or the necessity or advantage of a resection.

Thus, Bryant[52] tells of a painter who wished his arm to be fixed in a straight position, and of a turner whose knee at his own request was permitted to stiffen at a right angle, as that position allowed him to turn his wheel.

3. Excision for Disease of the Joint.—In our cold climate, so cursed by scrofula, and specially among the children of the labouring poor, such joint diseases are very prevalent, and whether the disease commences in the synovial membrane, the articular cartilages, or the heads of the bones, it frequently so disorganises the joint as to make it a question whether something must not be done to preserve the very life of the patient.

The difficulty of diagnosing the cases in which excisions are suitable or necessary is often very great; and we must balance its performance—(1.) against the possibly good results of an expectant treatment; (2.) against amputation of the limb.

(1.) Against expectant Treatment.—The patient has youth on his side, could we give him fresh sea air, good diet, cod oil, etc., we might very likely obtain anchylosis; true, but he may die while trying for this

---

[52] On Diseases and Injuries of Joints, p. 121.

anchylosis, and also this anchylosis, when got, may so lame or deform him that resection may still be required.

These points must all be considered, but as a general rule, I would say that such attempts at preservation of the limb are much more justifiable, and longer justifiable in the hip and knee-joints than in the elbow or shoulder; for the results in the lower limb will probably be as good, if the patient survive, if not better, than those obtained by excision, while the danger of the operation is greater; while in the upper limb, the danger to life in operating is less than that of leaving the limb on, and the results obtained by a successful operation, with well-managed after treatment, are far more satisfactory than the best possible anchylosis.

Another point bearing on this, of very great importance: In children, the most frequent subjects of such disease, excision of the lower limb may, by removing the epiphyses, cause to a very considerable degree disparity in their length, thus rendering them nearly useless, while in the upper such disparity is neither so extensive nor so injurious to the usefulness of the limb, which is not required for purposes of progression.

In the hip-joint especially, all the resources of the art should be tried in the expectant treatment, for amputation at the hip-joint is hardly ever admissible for disease of the joint, while excision has anything but satisfactory statistics.

(2.) Against Amputation.—Many questions must be considered, chiefly under the heads of the separate joints:—

1. As to the difficulties and dangers of the operations contrasted. Such as the following:—

Excisions give the surgeon more trouble, require more manual dexterity; take longer to perform; are very painful operations. Not valid objections in these days of chloroform and operative surgery on the dead body.

Excisions have the special peculiarity and danger of dealing chiefly with cancellated bone, broadened out, open, with numerous patulous canals for large veins, tending on any irritation or inflammation to set up a diffuse suppuration, and to culminate in phlebitis, myelitis, and other pyæmic conditions.

Excisions are performed through degenerate or disorganised, amputations through healthy, tissue.

Excisions require extreme care and absolute rest (i.e. in lower limb) for many weeks and months after the operation.

But, on the other hand,—

Amputations remove a portion of the body; excisions a much less one. Amputations are always necessarily nearer the centre than the corresponding excisions, and statistics show that the fatality of operations increases in exact proportion as they approach the centre.

77

A successful excision, especially in arm, saves a limb nearly perfect; an amputation at best is only the stump for a wooden one.

On the whole, there is actually very little difference in the mortality of excisions and amputations.

2. As to the results of the operation on the usefulness of the limb, depending on joint involved, age of patient, and amount of bone removed:—

A. *Joint involved.*—These must be noticed separately, but one thing is absolutely certain, that a much higher standard of usefulness, both in equality of length, amount of anchylosis, and position, is needed in the lower than in the upper limb. For a leg hanging like a flail, or shortened by some inches, is not so good for purposes of locomotion as a wooden leg is, while an arm, even though powerless at the elbow, and perhaps much shortened, can be so strengthened and supported by slings and bandages as to give a most useful hand, the complex movements and uses of the fingers of which no mechanism can at all imitate.

B. *Age of Patient.*—It must be remembered that excision in a child removes the epiphyses by which in great measure the growth of the bone is to be managed, and the stunted limb, especially in the leg, will eventually be of little advantage, though after the operation it looked excellently well, if a few years later it be found to be seven or eight inches shorter than its neighbour.

C. *Amount of Bone removed.*—From an erroneous view of the pathological changes in the bone affected, far too much was removed by many of the earlier operators, especially Moreau and Crampton.

The reason that this is often still the case, is well seen in many preparations. The bones are thickened to a considerable distance, and covered with irregular warty excrescences. These, which used to be considered evidences of disease, are only compact new healthy bone, thrown out like the callus of a fracture in consequence of the irritation.

In a word, what we require to remove is the following:—

1. All the cartilage, dead or alive, healthy or diseased.

2. Only the bone involving the articular extremities, in thin slices, or with the occasional use of the gouge, till a healthy bleeding surface is obtained.

3. The synovial membrane, however gelatinous or thickened looking, really requires very little care or notice; it will disappear of itself, partly by sloughing, partly by absorption during the profuse suppuration.[53]

Excision of the Shoulder-Joint.—Before considering the method

---

[53] For a very large amount of most interesting and valuable information on the whole subject of excisions of joints, I would refer to Dr. Hodge's most excellent work on this subject—On Excisions of Joints. By Richard M. Hodge, M.D., Boston, Massachusetts.

of operating, a word or two is required on the subject of how much is to be removed, and in what cases the operation should be performed. The shoulder and hip joints are the only ones in which partial excision is ever admissible, indeed, in the shoulder excision of the head of the humerus only is in many cases found to be all that is necessary, while in all it is much less dangerous to life than when the glenoid cavity also requires to be interfered with.

It is rarely necessary to remove more of the bone than merely its articular extremity (when performed for disease of the joint), and if possible this should be done inside the capsule, i.e. through an incision in the capsule, but without involving its attachment to the neck of the bone. When the glenoid is also diseased, mere gouging or scraping the cartilaginous surface will not suffice, but the neck must be thoroughly exposed, so that the whole cup of the glenoid may be removed by powerful forceps.

Cases suitable for Excision.—Cases of chronic disease of the head of the humerus (generally tubercular), or of chronic ulceration of the cartilages which has resisted counter-irritation. Cases of gunshot injury of the joint, or of compound dislocation, or fracture involving the joint. Cases of limited tumours affecting merely the head and upper third of the bone, and non-malignant in character. Anchylosis very rarely requires and would not be much benefited by such an operation.

Operation.—Though perhaps not the easiest, the following method is the one followed by the best results. It is suited especially for cases of caries or other disease of the joint, where the head of the humerus is either alone or chiefly affected:—

A single straight incision (Plate I. fig. a.) is made from a point just external to the coracoid process downwards along the humerus for at least three inches. It corresponds almost exactly to the bicipital groove, and has the advantage of avoiding the great vessels and nerves. The long head of the biceps may then be raised from its groove, and drawn to a side so as to be preserved. This is deemed of importance by Langenbeck and others. Mr. Syme, however, did not attach much value to its preservation, as it is often diseased. The capsule, which is often much altered, perhaps in part destroyed, is then opened, and the tendons of the muscles which rotate the head of the humerus divided in succession, while the elbow is rotated first inwards and then outwards by an assistant so as to put them on the stretch. The arm being then forced backwards, the head of the bone can be protruded through the wound, and sawn off at the necessary distance down the shaft. The glenoid must then be carefully examined, and any diseased bone removed by the cutting pliers. One or two small branches supplying the anterior fold of the axilla are the only vessels divided, and may not even require ligature, unless, indeed, from necrosis, or to remove a tumour, a larger portion of the humerus than usual has been removed. If the limit of capsule has been infringed on below, the circumflex vessels may probably be cut, in which case the bleeding may be considerable.

N.B.—In cases of fracture of neck of humerus, or of compound gunshot injury, or where the head has been separated by necrosis from the shaft, or where, as has happened to Stanley and others, the bone broke in the endeavour to tilt the head out, the surgeon will require to seize the detached head with strong forceps, and dissect it out with care.

Other methods of Resection.—When from great thickening and induration of the soft parts, enlargement of the head of the bone, or other reason, the straight incision may be deemed insufficient for the purpose (and we may remark that there are comparatively few cases in which it is insufficient), access may be obtained to the joint by raising a flap from the deltoid (Plate III. fig. a). Its shape—V-shaped, semilunar, or ovoid—is not of much consequence, for there are no great nerves or vessels to wound on the outside of the joint, and the surgeon should be guided, as in all other operations on the joint, very much by the position of any pre-existing sinuses. This flap being raised upwards towards its base, very free access is gained to the joint.

In these cases, fortunately comparatively rare, in which there is reason to believe that the glenoid is chiefly involved in disease, and yet that the disease can be removed without amputation, access will be gained most easily by an incision (Plate III. fig. b.) on the posterior surface of the joint, corresponding in size and direction to the linear incision in front. This gives a much easier mode of access to the glenoid. I have seen this practised in one very remarkable case by Mr. Syme, in which the glenoid cavity and neck of the scapula were extensively diseased, while the head of the bone was quite sound.

After-treatment is exceedingly simple; for the first day or two the shoulder is to be supported on a pillow with a simple pad in the axilla, if there is any tendency for the arm to drag inwards; after this the patient should be encouraged to sit up and move about with his arm in a sling, the elbow hanging freely down.

Results.—Hodge records ninety-six cases in which this excision was performed for gunshot injury, of which twenty-five proved fatal, and fifty for disease, of which only eight died,—results which are more encouraging than those of amputation at the shoulder-joint for disease; though for injury the mortality is much greater than Larrey's famous Statistics of Amputation, q.v. p. 65.

Spence had thirty-three cases, with three deaths. He generally made a counter-opening behind to get rid of discharges, and inserted a drainage-tube.

Gurlt's statistics of excision for gunshot injury give of 1661 cases 1067 recoveries, 27 doubtful results, and 567 deaths, the mortality being 34.70 per cent.

EXCISION OF THE ELBOW-JOINT—In what cases should it be

performed?—1. For disease of the elbow-joint which has resisted ordinary remedies, and is wearing down the patient's strength, including caries, ulceration of cartilages, and gelatinous synovial degeneration.

2. For wounds of the elbow penetrating the joint, the prognosis both as to the patient's life and the usefulness of his arm is much better after excision than after endeavours to save the joint without excision. This is especially the case when the wound of the joint is small and punctured, but if the case is seen early and treated by free drainage, with antiseptic precautions, excision may not be required.

3. For anchylosis, in cases where after disease or injury the limb has stiffened in a bad position, especially when, with a straight elbow, the hand is rendered almost perfectly useless.

How much should be removed?—In the elbow-joint, more than any other joint in the body, complete excision is absolutely necessary; any portion of the articular surface being left proves a source of unfavourable result.

The surgeon is apt to err rather in removing too little than too much. For the removal of too little bone is, on the one hand, apt to result in long-standing sinuses, on the other, to induce anchylosis.

In making the section of the bones, the saw ought to be applied to the humerus transversely just at the commencement of its condyloid projections, and to the radius and ulna, at least at a level with the base of the coronoid process of the ulna.

But while removing enough, we must not be led into the error of removing too much. If this is done, as was done by Sir Philip Crampton in his first case, and as happens occasionally of necessity in cases of excision for gunshot wounds or other accidents, much of the power of the arm is lost as a consequence of the shortening and excessive mobility.

A mistaken pathology sometimes deceives in the examination of the state of the bones, and causes an unnecessary amount to be removed. For in many cases of disease the bones in the neighbourhood of the joint are stimulated to an excessive amount of what is in reality Nature's effort at repair, and while the cartilaginous surfaces are denuded of cartilage, soft, and porous, the bones close by are roughened with a stalactitic-looking growth, projecting in knobs and angles. Now, if this be mistaken for disease and removed, too much will almost certainly be taken away, and the result will be unsatisfactory.

Much less care need be taken exactly to discriminate and remove the diseased soft parts; indeed they may be left alone; the synovial membrane in a state of gelatinous degeneration sometimes presents a very formidable appearance of disease, but if the bones be properly removed, all this swelling will soon go down, and a healthy condition of parts succeed, without any clipping or paring on the surgeon's part.

Operation.—The back of the joint is of course chosen for the seat

81

of the incisions, both because the bones are there just under the skin, and because the great vessels and nerves lie in front of the joint. The form and number of the incisions vary considerably, and ought to vary according to the nature of the case and the amount of disease or injury.

Though it is now little used, for historical interest I retain the description of the H-shaped incision (Plate III. fig. c.), used first by Moreau, and re-introduced by Mr. Syme, and used by him for most of his very numerous cases.

The posterior surface of the joint being exposed, the surgeon, with a strong straight bistoury, makes a transverse incision into the joint just above the olecranon. It should begin just far enough outside of the internal condyle to avoid the ulnar nerve, which the surgeon should protect by the forefinger of his left hand, and should extend transversely across to the outer condyle. From each end of this incision the surgeon should next make at a right angle two incisions, each about one inch and a half or two inches long, right down to the bone, thus marking out two quadrilateral flaps. These should next be raised from the bones, up and down, as much of the soft parts being retained in them as possible, so as to add to their thickness. The olecranon is thus exposed, and should be removed by saw or pliers by cutting into the greater sigmoid notch; the lateral ligaments must then be cut, if they are not already destroyed by the disease, and the humerus protruded, a proper amount of which is then to be sawn off in a transverse direction. The head of the radius is then easily removed by the bone-pliers, and the ulna also protruded, the attachment of the brachialis anticus to the coronoid process divided, and the bone sawn across just at the base of that process.

Few vessels, if any, will require ligature, and the arm being bent to nearly a right angle, the transverse incision must be very carefully sewed up with silver sutures closely set and deeply placed, as much of the future success of the joint depends on the completeness of the primary union of this incision. The external incision may also be accurately adjusted, the internal one not so completely, to allow free vent for the discharge, which is aided by the ligatures, if any are required, being brought out at its lower angle. A figure-of-8 bandage should be applied over pads of dry lint, and the limb laid on a pillow. No splint is necessary; in a few days the patient will be able to rise and walk about.

Passive motion should be begun so soon as the first inflammatory symptoms have passed off.

If properly performed, in a tolerably healthy subject, the surgeon should not be satisfied with any results short of almost perfect restoration of motion in the joint. Flexion and extension to their full extent, with a very considerable amount of pronation and supination, are to be expected, with proper care, in a patient of average intelligence.

Numerous cases are now on record where almost perfect performance of all the duties of life was retained after excision of the elbow-joint.[54]

In most cases it is possible, and in nearly all advisable, to excise the joint by means of a less complicated incision. Thus one long vertical incision at the posterior surface, with its centre about midway between the ulna and the external condyle, with a transverse incision at right angles to it, and reaching almost to the internal condyle, has been often practised with a very good result.

By nearly universal consent this single straight incision is now used, and when it is properly dressed and drained gives admirable results.

A single vertical incision (Plate III. fig. d.) without any transverse one, as long ago recommended by Chassaignac, is, in most cases, quite sufficient to give access. It is most suitable in cases of anchylosis, where there is little deposit of new bone, or in cases of disease of the joint, accompanied with little swelling or thickening of surrounding tissues. It has the advantage of avoiding the cicatrix of a transverse incision, which doubtless may, if at all a broad one, somewhat interfere with the future flexion of the limb, but, on the other hand, unless care is taken, it does not give such free egress for the discharge, and when there is much delay in healing, the vertical incision may leave a cicatrix nearly as troublesome as the other.

The following modification, suggested and practised by the late Mr. Maunder, seems to be a step in the right direction when it is practicable. "After a longitudinal incision crossing the point of the olecranon I next let the knife sink into the triceps muscle, and divide it longitudinally into two portions, the inner one of which is the more firmly attached to the ulna, while the outer portion is continuous with the anconeus muscle, and sends some tendinous fibres to blend with the fascia of the fore-arm. It is these latter fibres that are to be scrupulously preserved.

"Two points have to be remembered: first, the ulnar nerve, often unseen, must be lifted from its bed, and carried over the internal condyle to a safe place, and then the outer portion of the triceps muscle with its tendinous prolongation, the fascia of the fore-arm and the anconeus muscle must be dissected up, as it were, in one piece, sufficiently to allow of its being temporarily carried out over the external condyle of the humerus."[55]

---

[54] See Syme's Observations on Clinical Surgery, pp. 55, 57; Hodge on Excision of Joints, p. 63.
[55] Maunder's Operative Surgery, 2d ed. p. 123.

This method aids in retaining the power of active extension of the elbow-joint.

Excision for osseous anchylosis in the extended position of the joint may be sometimes rendered very difficult by the density, firmness, and extensive hypertrophy of the bones, which become fused into one solid mass. Any attempt to isolate the bones, and remove the anchylosed joint entire, by incising the bones as if for disease, will both prove very laborious, and also probably end in doing some damage to the vessels and nerves in front. But by sawing through the anchylosis about its centre, as was pointed out many years ago by Mr. Syme, the fore-arm may be flexed, and the bones as easily displayed, cleaned, and removed, as in the operation for disease. In this operation, as there is less thickening of the skin and subjacent textures, and in consequence more risk of deficiency and even sloughing of the flaps made by the H-shaped incision, a single straight incision will serve the purpose admirably.

Partial incisions of the elbow-joint are, as a rule, less successful and more dangerous to life than complete ones, except in cases of excision for anchylosis. Even in gunshot wounds, where the bones were previously healthy, and where uninjured portions might have been left with some hopes of success, this is the case.

Dr. Heron Watson has devised the following operation for cases of anchylosis the result of injury:—(1.) A linear incision over ulnar nerve at inner side of olecranon. (2.) The ulnar nerve to be carefully turned over the inner condyle. (3.) A probe-pointed bistoury to be introduced into the elbow-joint in front of the humerus, and then behind and carried upwards, so as to divide the upper capsular attachments in front and behind. (4.) A pair of bone-forceps to be next employed to cut off the entire inner condyle and trochlea of the humerus, and then introduced in the opposite diagonal direction so as to detach the external condyle and capitulum of the humerus from the shaft. (5.) The truncated and angular end of the humerus to be divided, turned out through the incision, and smoothed across at right angles to the line of the shaft by means of the saw, whereby (6.) room might be afforded, so that partly by twisting and partly by dissection the external condyle and capitulum are removed without any division of the skin on the outer side of the arm.[56] Six cases have had satisfactory results.

The mortality from this operation is considerably less than that from amputation of the arm. Of a series of excisions for disease, injury, and anchylosis, 22.15 per cent. died, while out of a similar series of amputations of the arm the mortality was 33.4 per cent.[57] Our mortality

[56] Edin. Med. Journal, May 1873.
[57] Quoted by Mr. Porter. Dublin Quarterly Journal for May 1867, p. 264.

of excision of the elbow here is certainly much less than the above. All of the cases, between thirty and forty, in which I have done it have recovered with but one exception, and Mr. Syme lost only one during the time I was his assistant.

Professor Spence lost only 16 in 189 cases, or 8.3 per cent.

Gurlt's statistics for gunshot injury give a mortality of over 24 per cent.

Out of 82 cases where the joint was excised for injury in the Schleswig-Holstein and Crimean campaigns, only 16 died; and out of 115 cases in which the joint was excised for disease, only 15 died.

The period after the injury at which the excision is performed seems to be important.

		Deaths	
Thus of 11 cases within	first twenty-four hours,	1	= 1-11
" 20 "	between second and fourth days,	4	= 1-5
" 9 " "	eighth and thirty-seventh,	1	= 1-9
40		6	

Excision of the Wrist.—Very various methods have been proposed and executed for the purpose of excising this joint. These vary much in difficulty and complexity, in proportion to the endeavours made to save the tendons from being cut.

The principles which must guide all attempts at operative interference with this joint are—

1. To remove all the diseased bone, including the cartilage-covered portions of the radius, ulna, and of the metacarpal bones, as little of these bones being removed as possible, beyond the cartilage-covered portions.

2. To disturb the tendons as little as possible, especially to avoid isolating them from the cellular sheath.

3. To commence passive motion of the fingers very soon after the operation.

It is rarely possible to remove the carpal bones as a whole, from the diseased condition which renders the operation necessary, and the digging out of the various bones piecemeal renders the operation very tedious, especially if the proximal ends of the metacarpal bones are involved and require to be removed, hence this operation was practically impossible till after the discovery of anæsthesia.

In describing the operation elaborated and described by Professor Lister, the type of the various plans in which the tendons are saved is given, while a very few words descriptive of the incisions used by others who cut the tendons will suffice.

LISTER'S OPERATION OF EXCISION OF THE WRIST-JOINT.—Even an abridgment of Mr. Lister's account of his operation must necessarily be long, because the operation itself is so complicated and prolonged, and guided by such precise principles, as to render much abridgment almost impossible.

A tourniquet is put on, to prevent oozing, which would conceal the state of the bones; any adhesions of the tendons must be then broken down by free movement of all the joints.

The radial incision (Plate IV. fig. a.) is then made. It commences at the middle of the dorsal aspect of the radius, on a level with the styloid process, passes as if going towards the inner side of the metacarpo-phalangeal joint of the thumb, in a line parallel to the extensor secundi internodii, but turns off at an angle as it passes the radial border of the second metacarpal, and then longitudinally downwards for half the length of that bone. The extensor carpi radialis brevior tendon is divided in the incision. The soft parts at the radial side are to be carefully dissected up, and the tendon of the extensor carpi radialis longior divided at its insertion. The cut tendons, and the extensor secundi internodii tendon and the radial artery can thus be pushed outwards, enabling the trapezium to be separated from the carpus by cutting-pliers. The extensor tendons being relaxed by bending back the hand, the soft parts must be cleared from the carpus as far as possible towards the ulnar side.

Fig. vi.[58]

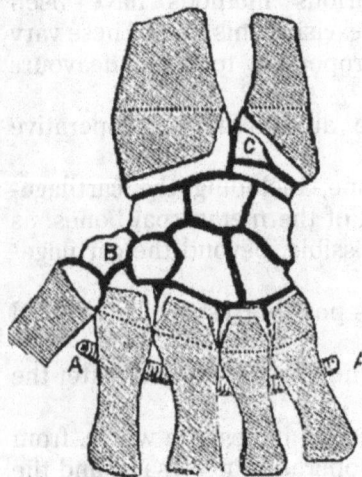

The ulnar incision (Plate IV. fig. b.) extends from two inches above the end of the ulna, in a line between the bone and the flexor carpi ulnaris, straight down as far as the middle of the palmar aspect of the fifth metacarpal. The dorsal lip of this incision is then raised, and the tendon of the extensor carpi ulnaris cut at its insertion, and reflected up out of its groove in the ulna along with the skin. The extensor tendons are then raised from the carpus, and the dorsal and lateral ligaments of the wrist divided, the tendons still being left as far as possible undisturbed in their relation to the radius. In front the

[58] A-A. Deep palmar arch; B. Trapezium; C. Articular surface of ulna; Dotted lines include the amount removed in Lister's earlier operations; Unshaded portions are those removed by Lister in cases where the disease is limited to the carpus. (Reduced from Lister's diagram in Lancet, 1865.)

flexor tendons are cleared from the carpus, the pisiform bone separated from the others though not removed, and the hook of the unciform divided by pliers. The knife must not go further down than the base of the metacarpal bones, in case of dividing the deep palmar arch. The anterior ligament of the wrist being now divided, the carpus and metacarpus are to be separated by cutting-pliers, and the carpus extracted by strong sequestrum forceps. By forcible eversion of the hand, the ends of radius and ulna can be protruded at the ulnar incision; as little as possible should be removed, consistent with removing all the disease. The ulna should be cut obliquely, leaving the base of the styloid process, and removing all the cartilage-covered portion. A thin slice of the radius is then to be cut also with the saw, so thin as to remove only the bevelled ungrooved portion, and leaving the tendons as far as possible undisturbed in their grooves. The ulnar articular facet is to be snipped off with bone-pliers. If the bones are more deeply carious, the diseased parts must at all hazards be removed with pliers or gouge. The metacarpal bones must then be treated in precisely the same way, their ends sawn off and their articular facets snipped off with the bone-pliers longitudinally. The trapezium is then to be seized by forceps and carefully dissected out, the metacarpal bone of the thumb pared like the others, the articular surface of the pisiform removed, the rest of the bone being left if it is sound. The radial incision is stitched closely throughout, and also the ends of the ulnar incision, any ligature being brought out through the centre of the ulnar incision, which is kept open with a piece of lint, which also gives support to the extensor tendons.

The after-treatment is important, the principal specialities being—(1.) early and free movement of the fingers; (2.) secure fixing of the wrist to procure consolidation. (1.) By passive motion of the joints of the knuckles and fingers, commenced on the second day, and continued daily after the operation; (2.) By a splint supporting the fore-arm and hand, the fingers being held in a semiflexed position by a large pad of cork fastened firmly on to the splint and made to fit the palm; this prevents the splint from slipping up the arm, and by a turn of a bandage insures fixation of the wrist-joint. The anterior part of this splint below the fingers may be gradually shortened, allowing more and more passive motion of the fingers, but the patient must wear it for months, indeed, till he finds his wrist as strong without it as with it.

Among the various operations that have been devised, the following require notice:—Mr. Spence, Dr. Gillespie, Dr. Watson, and the author, use a single dorsal incision with excellent results, and find it quite easy to remove all the bones from it. Mr. Spence had sixteen cases without a death.

POSTERIOR SEMILUNAR FLAP, from carpal attachment of metacarpal of index finger round to styloid process of ulna; dividing integuments only, then separating the tendons of the common extensor longitudinally, and drawing them aside by blunt hooks, the diseased bones are removed piecemeal by curved parrot-bill forceps.[59]

Posterior Curved Flap.—An incision down to the carpal bones, extended from a point two lines to the ulnar side of the extensor secundi internodii pollicis, and from a quarter to half an inch below the radio-carpal articulation, swept in a curvilinear direction downwards, close to the carpal extremities of the metacarpal bones, to a point just below the end of the ulna. The flap thus marked out was dissected up, and consisted of the integuments, areolar tissue, and extensor tendons of the four fingers, together with large deposits of fibrine, the products of repeated and prolonged inflammatory action. The tendon of the second extensor and its soft parts around were separated from the bones. The remains of the ligaments were cut, flexion of the hand protruded the carious ends of radius and ulna. The bones were then dissected out, leaving the trapezium, which was not diseased, and hand placed on a splint.[60]

EXCISION OF THE HIP-JOINT.—The question as to the propriety of performing this operation in any case is still debated by some surgeons, and the selection of suitable cases for the operation is greatly modified by the varying opinions of the different schools of surgery. Enough here to describe the method of operating, and the amount of the bone which is to be removed.

As in the shoulder-joint, the head of the femur is much more liable to disease, and, as a rule, much earlier attacked than is the acetabulum, but unfortunately the acetabulum does eventually become affected also in probably a much larger proportionate number of cases than the glenoid. Caries of the head, neck, and trochanters of the femur is a very common disease in this variable climate, and frequently connected with the strumous taint. After much suffering, abscesses form and discharge, giving considerable pain, and often end by carrying off the patient. As a result of the abscess and destruction of the ligaments, the head of the bone is apt to be displaced, and under some sudden muscular exertion or involuntary spasm, consecutive dislocation of the femur (generally on to the dorsum ilii) very often occurs.

In such a case the operation of excision of the head of the femur is by no means difficult, and not excessively dangerous, especially in young children.

Operation.—It is hardly necessary, or indeed possible, to lay down exact rules for the performance of this operation, in so far as the

59 Skey, Op. Surg., 2d ed. p. 438.
60 Abridged from Butcher, Op. and Con. Surgery, p. 208.

external incisions are concerned, for the sinuses which exist ought in general to be made use of.

When the surgeon has his choice, a straight incision (Plate II. fig. a.), parallel with the bone, extending from the top of the great trochanter downwards for about two inches, and also from the same point in a curved direction with the concavity forwards, upwards towards the position of the head of the bone (see diagram), will be found most convenient. The incisions should be carried boldly down to the bone, which will often be felt exposed and bathed in pus, any remains of the ligamentous structures must be cautiously divided with a probe-pointed bistoury, and then by bringing the knee of the affected side forcibly across the opposite thigh, with the toes everted, the head of the bone is forced out of the wound. The head, neck, and great trochanter should be fully exposed, and the saw applied transversely below the level of the trochanter, so as to remove it entire. If this is not done, it prevents discharge, protrudes at the wound, and besides this it is almost invariably diseased along with the head. Chain saws are quite unnecessary, it being in most cases easy to apply an ordinary one to the bone, if it is properly everted.

Great care in the after-treatment is required to prevent undue shortening of the limb, or in the event of a cure to secure the most favourable position for the anchylosis. The femur occasionally tends to protrude at the wound, and hence may require to be counter-extended by splints. If required at all, the splint should be made with an iron elbow opposite the wound to admit of its being easily dressed. In most cases counter-extension may be best managed by a weight and pulley.

Various forms of hammock swings to support the whole body, and slings of leather or canvas to support the limb only, have been found to aid recovery, and render the patient much more comfortable.

When the acetabulum is also diseased the prognosis is much more unfavourable than when it is sound.

The experiments of Heine and Jäger on the dead body, and operations by Hancock, Erichsen, and Holmes, on patients, have shown that in cases of extensive disease of the acetabulum it is quite possible by a prolonged and careful dissection to remove it all without injury of the pelvic viscera.

The details of incisions for such an operation need scarcely be given, as they must vary in each case with the amount of bone diseased, and the position of the already existing sinuses. The amount of bone that may be removed varies much. Erichsen in one case excised "the upper end of the femur, the acetabulum, the rami of the pubis, and of the ischium, a portion of the tuber ischii, and part of the dorsum ilii."[61]

A less formidable proceeding may be useful in cases where the

---

[61] Science and Art of Surgery, 3d ed. p. 745.

acetabulum is diseased, but not deeply. The moderate use of an ordinary gouge may succeed in removing the diseased bone.

Experience and the cold evidence of statistics prove, however, that the prognosis in any case is modified very much for the worse by the presence of any disease of the acetabulum, more than one-half of the cases proving fatal in which it is diseased, whether attempts to remove the disease of the acetabulum be made or not, and that those cases do best in which the head of the femur has been displaced, and lies outside the joint almost like a loose sequestrum among the soft parts.

The results of excision of the hip have as yet been very discouraging, the mortality of the whole series of published cases being, according to Dr. Hodge's careful table, very little under 1 in every 2 cases, viz., 1 in 2-5/53. Later statistics are however more favourable.

Like all other excisions, the mortality increases very much with the patient's age.

Thus of 103 completed cases in which the age is given, 53 recovered and 50 died, but dividing the cases at the end of the sixteenth year, we find that of the children below this age 43 recovered and 29 died, a mortality of 40.2 per cent.; of the adults, 10 recovered, and 21 died, or a mortality of 67.6 per cent.

If we remember the marvellous power of recovery from joint diseases we find in childhood, under the influence of good diet, cod-liver oil, and fresh air, we cannot shut our eyes to the fact that such results and such a mortality are by no means encouraging.

From an extensive experience in a special hospital for hip-disease, where fresh air, abundant nourishment, and very excellent nursing are provided, the author is learning more and more to trust to the power of nature in the cure of even very advanced cases of hip-disease in children, and he believes that operation is rarely necessary, or even warrantable, except for the removal of sequestra.

Mr. Holmes's[62] statistics are interesting. He has operated on no fewer than nineteen cases. Of these seven died, one after secondary amputation at the hip. Another required amputation and recovered. Two others died of other diseases without having used their limb. Of the remaining nine, three were perfectly successful, four were promising cases, and two unpromising.

Professor Spence in 19 cases had 6 deaths, or a mortality of 31.6 per cent.

Culbertson's collection gives out of 426 cases, 192 deaths, or 45 per cent.

Mr. Croft, whose skill and success as an operator are well known, has recorded 45 cases of excision of hip in his own practice; of these 16 died, 11 were under treatment, 18 had

---

[62] On the Surgical Treatment of Children's Diseases, pp. 454-6.

recovered, of which 16 had moveable joints and useful limb; the other two are "potentially cured."[63]

Various other incisions have been devised for gaining access to the joint. The most noticeable are those in which a flap is made instead of a linear incision. Sedillot makes a semilunar or ovoid flap, the base of which is just below the great trochanter, and which includes it, the convexity being upwards and the flap being turned down. Gross's modification of this is preferable, being turned the opposite way, the convexity being downwards (Plate III. fig. e.), and the flap thus being turned up.

Results in successful cases.—Of fifty-two in Hodge's table, thirty-one had useful limbs, six indifferent, three decidedly useless, four died within three years, and of the remaining eight no details are given.

The shortening is always considerable, a high-heeled shoe being required in most cases; a stick is indispensable; in many, crutches are necessary.

Various operations have been devised for the treatment of osseous anchylosis of the hip-joint when in a bad position. All are more or less dangerous. Perhaps one of the least dangerous is the plan of subcutaneous division of the neck of the femur by a narrow saw, proposed by Mr. Adams of London. It is sometimes a very laborious operation.

Excision of Knee-Joint.—Removal of Bone.—In every case the excision of the joint ought to be complete. Some attempts have been made to save one or other of the articular surfaces, but they have proved failures. The patella has frequently been left when it was not diseased, as is often the case, but the results have not been such as to recommend such a practice.

Direction of Section of the Bones.—The bones should be cut transversely, and, as far as possible, be in accurate and complete apposition. A slight bevelling at the expense of the posterior margin will produce an anchylosis of the limb in a very slightly flexed position, which is found to aid the patient in walking.

It has been proposed by some[64] to cut both bones obliquely, so as to obviate the difficulty of making the transverse surfaces parallel. This involves a still greater practical difficulty in keeping these oblique surfaces in position during the after-treatment.

This plan might possibly be valuable in cases where the disease was limited to one or other edge of the bone.

Among the various incisions recommended, the best seems to be the Semilunar Incision.

Operation.—The limb being held in an extended position, a

---

[63] Clinical Society's Transactions, vol. xiii. p. 71.
[64] Billroth of Vienna and Pelikan of St. Petersburg, quoted from Heyfelder by Hodge on Excision of Joints, p. 161.

single semilunar incision (Plate I. fig. b.) is made, entering the joint at once, and dividing the ligamentum patellæ. It should extend from the inner side of the inner condyle of the femur to a corresponding point over the outer one, passing in front of the joint midway between the lower edge of the patella and tuberosity of the tibia. The flap is then dissected back, the ligaments divided, when by extreme flexion of the limb the articular surface of the tibia and femur are thoroughly exposed. The crucial ligaments must then be divided cautiously, and the articular portion of the femur cleaned anteriorly by the knife, posteriorly by the operator's finger, so far as possible to avoid injury of the artery. The whole articular surface of the femur must then be removed by a transverse cut with the saw as exactly as possible at a right angle with the axis of the bone. The amount of the femur which will require removal will in the adult vary from an inch to an inch and a half or even more. It must involve all the bone normally covered by cartilage; and this being removed, if the section shows evidence of disease, slice after slice may require removal till a healthy surface is obtained. Occasionally, if the diseased portion appears limited, though deep, the application of a gouge may succeed in removing disease without involving too great shortening of the limb. Specially in children, it is of great importance to avoid removing the whole epiphysis. The tibia must then be exposed in a similar manner, and a thin slice removed; if the bone be tolerably healthy, even less than half an inch will prove quite sufficient.

This method has an immense advantage in that it provides an excellent anterior flap for the amputation, which may be required in cases where the disease of bone is found too extensive to admit of the excision being practised.

This method, with slight deviations, is substantially that of Richard Mackenzie of Edinburgh, Wood of New York, Jones of Jersey.

Hæmorrhage must then be stopped, and that as thoroughly as possible, by torsion, cold, and pressure, and the flap brought accurately together with sutures.

In some rare cases, it may be found necessary to divide the hamstring tendons to rectify spastic contraction of the muscles; but this can generally be done quite well from the original wound.

Holt makes a dependent opening in the popliteal space for drainage. This is unnecessary if the incisions are made sufficiently far back, and if the wound is properly drained. It is unsafe, as approaching so close to the artery and veins. If much bagging takes place, the use of a drainage-tube will prove quite sufficient.

After-treatment.—Wire splints lined with leather and provided with a foot-piece; special box-splints with moveable sides, as Butcher's;[65] plaster-of-Paris moulds are used by Dr. P.H. Watson[66] of

---

[65] Operative and Conservative Surgery, pp. 28, 138.

Edinburgh and others; this last form of dressing is the best, and allows the limb to be suspended from a Salter's swing.

H-shaped incision.—The internal incision should commence at a point about two inches below the articular surface of the tibia, and in a line with its inner edge; it should then be carried up along the femur in a direction parallel to the axis of the extended limb, so as to pass in front of the saphena vein, and thus avoid it, for a distance of five inches. The external incision, commencing just below the head of the fibula, must be carried upwards parallel to the preceding for the same distance. Both incisions must be made by a heavy scalpel with a firm hand, so as to divide all the tissues down to the bone. The vertical incisions are then united by a transverse one passing across just below the lower angle of the patella. The flaps thus formed must then be dissected up and down, and the internal and external lateral ligaments divided, thus thoroughly opening the joint and exposing the crucial ligaments. These must be divided carefully, remembering the position of the artery. The bones are then to be cleared and divided, as in the operation already described. This is the method of Moreau and Butcher.[66]

Patella and Ligamentum Patellæ retained.—"A longitudinal incision, full four inches in extent, was made on each side of the knee-joint, midway between the vasti and flexors of the leg; these two cuts were down to the bones, they were connected by a transverse one just over the prominence of the tubercle of the tibia, care being taken to avoid cutting by this incision the ligamentum patellæ; the flap thus defined was reflected upwards, the patella and the ligament were then freed and drawn over the internal condyle, and kept there by means of a broad, flat, and turned-up spatula; the joint was thus exposed, and after the synovial capsule had been cut through as far as could be seen, the leg was forcibly flexed, the crucial ligaments, almost breaking in the act, only required a slight touch of the knife to divide them completely. The articular surfaces of the bones were now completely brought to view, and the diseased portions removed by means of suitable saws, the soft parts being hold aside by assistants."[68]

Results of Excision of Knee-joint:—Holmes's Table of recent cases from 1873-1878—

	245 cases;	25 deaths, and 47 failures.
Spence's	33 cases;	22 recovered, 11 died.

Buck's Operation for Anchylosed Knee-Joint.—The principle of this operation is to remove a triangular portion of bone, which is to include the surfaces of the femur and tibia, which have anchylosed in

---

[66] On Excision of Knee-Joint, pp. 18, 20.
[67] Operative and Conservative Surgery, p. 169.
[68] Mr. Jones of Jersey, Med. Chir. Trans., vol. xxxvii. p. 68.

an awkward position, and by this means to set the bones free, and enable the limb to be straightened. Access to the joint may be obtained by either of the two methods already described. Sections of the bones are then to be made with the saw, so as to meet posteriorly a little in front of the posterior surface of the anchylosed joint, and thus remove a triangular portion of bone; the portion still remaining, and which still keeps up the deformity, is then to be broken through as best you can, either by a chisel, or a saw, or forced flexion. The ends are to be pared off by bone-pliers, and the surfaces brought into as close apposition as possible. The operation is a difficult one, a gap being generally left between the anterior edges of the bones, from the unyielding nature of the integuments behind, and the difficulty of removing the posterior projecting edges from their close proximity to the artery. Of twenty cases on record, eight died, and two required amputation.

Relation of Age to result in Excision of Knee-Joint from Hodge's Tables.

Of 182 complete cases:—

68 below 16 years: 50 recovered—18 died; or 26 per cent. died.
114 above 16 years: 55 recovered—59 died; or 51.7 per cent. died.

EXCISION OF THE ANKLE-JOINT.—*In what cases is it to be done, and how much bone is to be removed?*

In cases of compound dislocation of the ankle-joint, the tibia and fibula are apt to be protruded either in front or behind. When this happens it is a dislocation generally very difficult to reduce, and when reduced to retain in position. In such cases, if there seems to be any chance of retaining the foot, excision of the articular ends of tibia and fibula greatly add to the probabilities in its favour. It may be done without any new wound, and, in general, by an ordinary surgeon's saw.

When the astragalus does not protrude, it seems to matter little for the future result whether its articular surface be removed or not. When, on the other hand, it protrudes, as a result either of the displacement of the entire foot, or of a dislocation complete or partial of the astragalus itself, there is no doubt that excision either of its articular surface or of the entire bone will give very excellent results. Jäger reports twenty-seven such cases, with only one fatal, and one doubtful result.

In cases of disease of the Ankle-joint.—Excision has been performed a good many times, and should in most cases be complete. A work like this is not the place to discuss the propriety of operations so much as the method of performing them, but one remark may be permitted. Few points of surgical diagnosis are more difficult than it is to tell whether in any given case disease is confined to the ankle-joint, and whether or not the bones of the tarsus participate. If they do even to a slight extent, no operation which attacks the ankle-joint only has any reasonable chance of success. It may look well for a time, but sinuses remain, the irritation of the operation only hastens the progress of the disease of the bone, and the result will almost certainly be disappointing, amputation being almost the inevitable dernier ressort.

Methods of Operating:—

Mr. Hancock has been very successful by the following method:—

Commence the incision (Plate II. figs. B.B.) about two inches above and behind the external malleolus, and carry it across the instep to about two inches above and behind the internal malleolus. Take care that this incision merely divides the skin, and does not penetrate beyond the fascia. Reflect the flap so made, and next cut down upon the external malleolus, carrying your knife close to the edge of the bone, both behind and below the process, dislodge the peronei tendons, and divide the external lateral ligaments of the joint. Having done this, with the bone-nippers cut through the fibula, about an inch above the malleolus, remove this piece of bone, dividing the inferior tibio-fibular ligament, and then turn the leg and foot on the outside. Now carefully dissect the tendons of the tibialis posticus and flexor communis digitorum from behind the internal malleolus. Carry your knife close round the edge of this process, and detach the internal lateral ligament, then grasping the heel with one hand, and the front of the foot with the other, forcibly turn the sole of the foot downwards, by which the lower end of the tibia is dislocated and protruded through the wound. This done, remove the diseased end of the tibia with the common amputating saw, and afterwards with a small metacarpal saw placed upon the back of the upper articulating process of the astragalus, between that process and the tendo Achillis, remove the former by cutting from behind forwards. Replace the parts in situ; close the wound carefully on the inner side and front of the ankle; but leave the outside open, that there may be a free exit for discharge, apply water-dressing, place the limb on its outer side on a splint, and the operation is completed.

Skin, external, and internal ligaments, and the bones are the only parts divided, no tendons and no arteries of any size.[69]

Barwell's method by lateral incisions is briefly as follows:—

On the outer side, an incision over the lower three inches of the fibula turns forward at the malleolus at an angle, and ends about half an inch above the base of the outer metatarsal. The flap is to be reflected, fibula divided about two inches from its lower end by the forceps, and dissected out, leaving peronei tendons uncut. A similar incision on the inner side terminates over the projection of the internal cuneiform bone; the sheaths of the tendons under inner angle are then to be divided, and the artery and nerve avoided; the internal lateral ligament is then to be divided, the foot twisted outwards, so as to protrude the astragalus and tibia at the inner wound. The lower end of

---

[69] Lancet, Oct. 1, 1859.

the tibia and top of the astragalus are to be sawn off by a narrow-bladed saw passing from one wound to the other.[70]

Dr. M. Buchanan of Glasgow has described an operation by which the joint can be excised through a single incision over the external malleolus.

Results.—So far as can be gathered from cases already published, the results are very often (at least in one out of every two cases) unsatisfactory. Sinuses remain, which do not heal, the limbs are useless, and amputation is in the end necessary.

Langenbeck has performed it sixteen times during the last Schleswig-Holstein war (in 1864), and the Bohemian war in 1866, with only three deaths. In these cases the operation was subperiosteal.

EXCISION OF THE SCAPULA.—More or less of the scapula has in many cases been removed along with the arm, and even with the addition of portion of the clavicle.

Excision of the entire bone, leaving the arm, has been performed in two instances by Mr. Syme. The procedure must vary according to the nature and shape of the tumour on account of which the operation is performed. Mr. Syme operated as follows:—

In the first case, one of cerebriform tumour of the bone, he "made an incision from the acromion process transversely to the posterior edge of the scapula, and another from the centre of this one directly downwards to the lower margin of the tumour. The flaps thus formed being reflected without much hæmorrhage, I separated the scapular attachment of the deltoid, and divided the connections of the acromial extremity of the clavicle. Then, wishing to command the subscapular artery, I divided it, with the effect of giving issue to a fearful gush of blood, but fortunately caught the vessel and tied it without any delay. I next cut into the joint and round the glenoid cavity, hooked my finger under the coracoid process, so as to facilitate the division of its muscular and ligamentous attachments, and then pulling back the bone with all the force of my left hand, separated its remaining attachments with rapid sweeps of the knife." (Plate III. fig. g.)

Mr. Syme's second case was also one of tumour of the scapula; the head of the humerus had been excised two years before.

He removed it by two incisions, one from the clavicle a little to the sternal side of the coracoid, directed downwards to the lower boundary of the tumour, another transversely from the shoulder to the posterior edge of the scapula. The clavicle was divided at the spot where it was exposed, and the outer portion removed along with the scapula.[71]

The author has in a case of osseous tumour removed the whole

---

[70] Barwell On Diseased Joints, p. 464.
[71] Syme On Excision of the Scapula, pp. 13-26, 1864.

body of the scapula, leaving glenoid, spine, acromion and anterior margin with excellent result and a useful arm.

Large portions of the shafts of the humerus, radius, and ulna have been removed for disease or accident, and useful arms have resulted; but as the operative procedures must vary in every case, according to the amount of bone to be removed, and the number and position of the sinuses, no exact directions can be given.

For very interesting cases of such resections reference may be made to Wagner's treatise on the subject, translated and enlarged by Mr. Holmes, and to Williamson's Military Surgery, p. 227.

Excision of Metacarpals and Phalanges.—To excise the metacarpal implies that the corresponding finger is left. Except in cases of necrosis, where abundance of new bone has formed in the detached periosteum, the results of such excisions do not encourage repetition, the digits which remain being generally very useless. It is quite different, however, if it is the thumb that is involved; and every effort should, in every case, be made to retain the thumb, even in the complete absence of its metacarpal bone. For the good results of a case in which Mr. Syme excised the whole metacarpal bone for a tumour, see his Observations in Clinical Surgery, p. 38.

The operation is not difficult, and requires merely a straight incision over the dorsum, extending the whole length of the bone.

In the same way the proximal phalanx of the thumb may be excised, and yet, if proper care be taken, a very useful limb be left. I quote entire the following case by Mr. Butcher of Dublin:—

Excision of Proximal Phalanx of the Thumb.—The thumb of the right hand was crushed by the crank of a steam-engine. The proximal phalanx was completely shivered; its fragments were removed, the cartilage of the proximal end of the distal phalanx, and also of the head of the metacarpal bone, were pared off with a strong knife. The digit was put up on a splint fully extended. In about a month cure was nearly complete, a firm dense tissue took the place of the removed phalanx, and the power of flexing the unguinal was nearly complete.[72]

Excision of the Joints of the Fingers.—These operations may be performed for compound dislocation, specially when the thumb is injured; no directions can be given for the incisions.[73]

In cases of disease it is rarely necessary or advisable to attempt to save a finger, but if the metacarpo-phalangeal joint of the thumb be affected, excision should be performed with the hope of saving the thumb. A single free incision on the radial side of the joint will give sufficient access.

EXCISION OF THE OS CALCIS.—In those comparatively rare cases in which the os calcis is alone affected, the rest of the tarsus and

---

[72] Butcher's Operative and Conservative Surgery, p. 225.
[73] For an excellent case, see Annandale on Diseases of the Finger and Toes, p. 261.

the ankle-joint being healthy, a considerable difference of opinion exists as to the proper course to be followed. By some surgeons it is considered best merely to gain free access to the diseased bone, and then remove by a gouge all the softened and altered portions, leaving a shell of bone all round, of course saving the periosteum and avoiding interference with the joint. This operation requires no special detailed instruction. We find many surgeons, among them Fergusson and Hodge, supporters of this comparatively modest operation. The author has many times performed this operation with excellent results. Even when nothing but periosteum is left, the new bone becomes strong and of full size.

Excision of the whole of the diseased bone at its joints, with or without an attempt to leave some of the periosteum, has been deemed necessary by others. Holmes, who has had considerable experience, removes the bone at once by the following incisions, without paying any reference to the periosteum:—

Operation.—An incision (Plate III. fig. f.) is commenced at the inner edge of the tendo Achillis, and drawn horizontally forwards along the outer side of the foot, somewhat in front of the calcaneo-cuboid joint, which lies midway between the outer malleolus and the end of the fifth metatarsal bone. This incision should go down at once upon the bone, so that the tendon should be felt to snap as the incision is commenced. It should be as nearly as possible on a level with the upper border of the os calcis, a point which the surgeon can determine, if the dorsum of the foot is in a natural state, by feeling the pit in which the extensor brevis digitorum arises. Another incision is then to be drawn vertically across the sole, commencing near the anterior end of the former incision, and terminating at the outer border of the grooved or internal surface of the os calcis, beyond which point it should not extend, for fear of wounding the posterior tibial vessels. If more room be required, this vertical incision may be prolonged a little upwards, so as to form a crucial incision. The bone being now denuded by throwing back the flaps, the first point is to find and lay open the calcaneo-cuboid joint, and then the joints with the astragalus. The close connections between these two bones constitute the principal difficulty in the operation on the dead subject; but these joints will frequently be found to have been destroyed in cases of disease. The calcaneum having been separated thus from its bony connections by the free use of the knife, aided, if necessary, by the lever, lion-forceps, etc., the soft parts are next to be cleaned off its inner side with care, in order to avoid the vessels, and the bone will then come away.[74]

Attempts may occasionally be made in such an operation to save a portion of periosteum in attachment to the soft parts, but success or failure in this seems to have very little effect on the future result.

---

[74] Holmes's Surgery, 3d edition, vol. iii. p. 771.

Hancock's Method.—A single flap was formed in the sole, with the convexity looking forwards, by an incision from one malleolus to the other.

Greenhow's Method.—Incisions made from the inner and outer ankles, meeting at the apex of the heel, and then others extending along the sides of the foot, the flaps being dissected back so as to expose the bone and its connections.[75]

EXCISION OF ASTRAGALUS.—A curved incision on the dorsum of the foot extending from one malleolus to the other, and as far forwards as the front of the scaphoid. The chief caution required is to divide all ligaments which hold the bone in place, and dissect it clean on all other parts before meddling with its posterior surface where the groove exists for the flexor longus pollicis tendon near which the posterior tibial vessels and nerve lie.[76]

EXCISION OF ASTRAGALUS AND SCAPHOID.—An incision similar to the anterior one in Syme's amputation at the ankle. The flap was then turned back from the dorsum of the foot. The joint was then opened, the lateral ligaments of the ankle-joint divided, the foot dislocated so as to show the astragalo-calcanean ligaments, and allow them to be divided. The bones were then grasped with the lion-forceps and pulled forwards, while the posterior surface of the astragalus was very cautiously cleaned, so as to avoid the posterior tibial artery.[77]

EXCISION OF METATARSO-PHALANGEAL JOINT OF GREAT TOE.—Butcher performs it by splitting up the sinuses leading to the carious joint, exposing it and cutting off with bone-pliers the anterior third of the metatarsal bone, and the proximal end of the first phalanx. He also cuts subcutaneously the extensor tendons to prevent them from cocking up the toe.[78] Pancoast prefers a semilunar incision. A lateral incision is usually to be preferred.

The author has performed this excision frequently for disease; when the whole cartilages are removed and the wound is freely drained, an admirable result is obtained.

In cases of compound dislocation of the head of the metatarsal bone, it will occasionally be found necessary to excise it either by the original, or a slightly enlarged wound.

The author lately excised one-half of shaft of metatarsal and the corresponding half of proximal phalanx of great toe for exostosis, with antiseptic precautions. The result was a useful toe with a mobile joint.

EXCISION OF METATARSAL BONE OF GREAT TOE.—For this operation a quadrilateral flap has been recommended, but this is quite unnecessary. A single straight incision along the inner border of the

---

[75] Brit. and Foreign Med. Chir. Review for July 1853.
[76] Mr. Holmes in Lancet for February 18, 1856.
[77] Ibid. for May 1865.
[78] Butcher, Operative and Conservative Surgery, p. 354.

foot, extending the whole length of the bone, renders it very easy to remove the whole bone from joint to joint. This is an operation, however, which is rarely needed, and which would leave a very useless flail of a toe. The operation, which is at once more commonly required, and also gives promise of a more satisfactory result, is the one performed for cario-necrosis of the shaft only, and in the following manner:—

A straight incision through all the tissues, including the periosteum, right down to the bone; then with nail or handle of the knife to separate the periosteum from the bone; then with a pair of bone-pliers or a fine saw to divide the shaft from both its extremities and remove it entire.[79]

[79] See Butcher, Operative and Conservative Surgery, p. 356.

CHAPTER IV

OPERATIONS ON CRANIUM AND SCALP

TREPHINING AND TREPANNING are the names given to operations for the removal of portions of the cranium by circular saws which play on a centre pivot. When the motion is given to the saw simply by rotation of the hand of the operator, as is common in this country, it is called trephining; when (as used to be the case in this country, and still is on the Continent) the motion is given by an instrument like a carpenter's brace, the operation is called trepanning.

The nature of the operation varies according to the nature of the case for which it is performed. Thus (1.) it may be performed through the uninjured cranium in the hope of evacuating an abscess of the diploe or dura mater, or of relieving pressure caused by suppuration in the brain itself, or by extravasation into the brain or membranes; or (2.) it may be required in cases of punctured and depressed fracture for the purpose of removing projecting corners of bone and allowing elevation of the depressed portions; or (3.) it is sometimes used to remove a circular portion of bone in cases of epilepsy in which pain or tenderness is felt at some limited portion of the cranium.

1. *In cases where the cranium and its coverings are entire.*— There are certain positions where, if it is possible, the trephine should not be applied. These are the longitudinal sinus, the anterior inferior angle of the parietal bone, where the middle meningeal artery is in the way, the occipital protuberance, and the various sutures. These being avoided, a crucial incision is to be made through the skin, and its flaps reflected. The pericranium should then be raised from the centre, for a space large enough to hold the crown of the trephine. The pericranium should never be removed, but carefully raised and preserved, as its presence will greatly aid in the restoration of bone.[80] The centre pin should then be projected for about the eighth of an inch and bored into the bone. On it as a centre the saw is then worked by semicircular sweeps in both directions alternately, till it forms a groove for itself. Whenever this groove is deep enough the pin should be retracted, lest from its projection it pierce the dura mater before the tables of the skull are cut through. Were the cranium always of the same thickness, and even of similar consistence, the operation would always be exceedingly easy; but in both these particulars different skulls vary much from each other, and thus by a rash use of the instrument the dura mater may possibly be injured. The tough outer table is more difficult to cut than

---

[80] See case by the author in the Edin. Med. Jour. for June 1868.

the softer and more vascular diploe, and the inner table is denser than either, but more brittle. In many old skulls, however, the diploe is wanting altogether, and the two tables are amalgamated, and often very thin.

Great care must be taken in every case to saw slowly, to remove the sawdust, and examine the track of the saw by a probe or quill, lest one part should be cut through quicker than another. The last turns of the instrument must specially be cautious ones. When the disk of bone does not at once come away in the trephine, the elevator or the special forceps for the purpose will easily remove it. If the abscess, extravasation, or exostosis be then discovered and removed, all that remains is to remove any sawdust or loose pieces of bone, and possibly to smooth off any sharp edges of the orifice by an instrument called the lenticular. This is very seldom required, and now hardly ever used.

2. *In cases of depressed or punctured fracture* the trephine is occasionally required (when symptoms of compression are present) for the purpose of enabling the depressed portion to be elevated. It is unsafe to apply it to the depressed or fractured bone, lest the additional pressure of the instrument should cause wound of the dura mater or brain. It is generally applied on some projecting corner of sound bone under which the depressed portion is locked, and hence it is rarely necessary to remove a complete circular portion. In fact very many cases of such displacement may be remedied more easily by a pair of strong bone-forceps, or a Hey's saw, applied to remove the projecting portion of sound bone. The same precautions must be used as in the operation already described, and the sawing must be done even more cautiously, as it is rarely more than a semicircle that requires cutting.

In former days trephining was a much more frequent operation than it is now, and apparently more successful. The reason of the greater apparent success can easily be found in the fact that it was performed in many cases merely as a precautionary measure against dreaded inflammation of the brain, which probably never would have appeared at all, and that the operation itself is one by no means dangerous. Very numerous applications of the trephine have been made in the same individual—two, four, six, and even in one case twenty-seven disks having been removed from the same skull, and yet the patients have survived.

TUMOURS OF THE SCALP, *Removal of.*—By far the most frequent are the encysted tumours, or wens. These consist of a thick firm cyst-wall, which contains soft, curdy, or pultaceous matter, sometimes almost fluid, at others dry and gritty. They are loosely attached in the subcutaneous cellular tissue, and unless they have become very large, or have been much pressed on, are non-adherent to the skin.

The treatment is thus very simple. They should merely be

transfixed by a sharp knife, the contents evacuated, and the cyst seized by strong dissecting forceps and twisted out.

If they have once become adherent, they must be dissected out in the usual manner, after the adherent portion of skin has been defined by elliptical incisions.

In the case of large wens on visible parts of scalp or face, the author avoids scar, by the following plan:—

Make a small incision, two lines at most, through skin only, then with a blunt probe separate the cyst from the skin subcutaneously; then, pulling it to the wound with catch-forceps, empty the cyst and gradually pull it out, as if taking out an ovarian cyst. No scar but a dimple will remain.

CHAPTER V

OPERATIONS ON EYE

Operations on the Eye and its Appendages

OPERATIONS ON THE LIDS.—

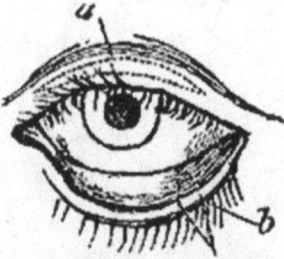

Fig. vii.[81]

1. FOR ENTROPIUM OR INVERSION OF THE LIDS, OFTEN COMBINED WITH TRICHIASIS, IRREGULARITY OF THE CILIÆ.—As in many cases the entropium seems to depend partly on a too great laxity of the skin of the lid, combined occasionally with spasm of the orbicularis, the simplest and most natural plan of operation is (a) to remove (Fig. vii. a) an elliptical portion of skin, extending transversely along the whole length of the affected lid, including the fibres of the orbicularis lying below it, and then to unite the edges with several points of fine suture. (b) An improvement on this in obstinate cases is proposed by Mr. Streatfeild (Fig. viii.) He continues the same incision, but in addition removes a long narrow wedge-shaped portion of the tarsal cartilage, grooving it without entirely cutting it through, in such a manner that the retraction of the skin bends the cartilage backwards, thus everting to a very considerable extent the previously inverted ciliæ.[82]

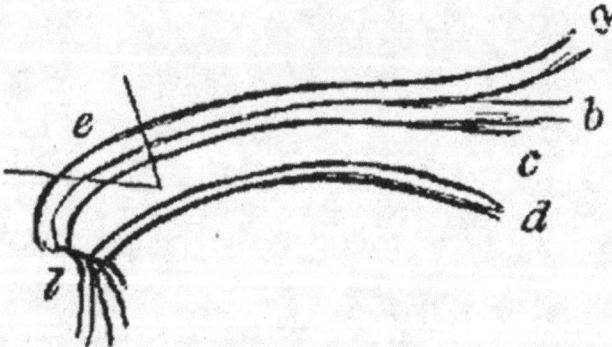

Fig. viii.

---

[81] a. Elliptical incision for entropium; b. wedge-shaped incision for ectropium.
[82] Ophthalmic Hospital Reports, vol. i. p. 121.

2. ECTROPIUM is the opposite condition from entropium; in it the eyelids are everted and the palpebral conjunctiva is exposed.

If the result of cicatrix, of a burn, or of disease of bone, the treatment must be varied according to circumstances, and in many cases, skin must be transplanted to fill the gap.

In the more usual cases resulting from chronic inflammation the following simple operations are required:—1. In mild cases the excision of an elliptical portion of conjunctiva may suffice, the edges must not be left to contract, but should be brought carefully together. 2. In more chronic cases, where all the tissues of the lid are very lax, it is necessary to remove (Fig. vii. b) a V-shaped portion of lid and skin, and then stitch it very carefully up with interrupted sutures.

TUMOURS OF EYELIDS.—1. *Encysted tumours; cysts of the lids; tarsal tumour.*—Under these and similar names are recognised a very frequent form of disease, chiefly in the upper lid: small tumours which rarely exceed half a pea in size, convex towards the skin, which is freely moveable over them; they give no pain, and are annoying only from their bulk and deformity.

Operation.—Evert the lid, incise the conjunctiva freely over the tumour, insert the blunt end of a probe and roughly stir up the contents of the cyst, thus evacuating it. If the tumour is large and of old standing it may be requisite to cut out an elliptical or circular portion of its conjunctival wall. The probe may require to be reapplied once or twice at intervals of two or three days, and in certain rare cases it may be necessary as a last resource freely to cauterise the inside of the cyst with the solid nitrate of silver.

In no case is it ever necessary to excise the tumour from the outside of the eyelid; when this has been done in error there frequently remains an awkward and unsightly scar.

2. *Fibrous cysts*, frequently congenital, are met with in one situation, just over the external angular process of the frontal bone. These are larger in size than the preceding, ranging from the size of a barley pickle to that of an almond. Their treatment is excision by a prolonged and careful dissection from the periosteum, to which they almost invariably are adherent.

OPERATIONS ON THE LACHRYMAL ORGANS.—In a system of ophthalmic surgery, various operative procedures might be detailed under this head, authorised and sanctioned by old custom. Excision of a diseased lachrymal gland, and removal of stones in the gland or ducts, need no special directions for their performance, and the operation immediately to be described, under the head of Mr. Bowman's operation, is applicable in almost every one of the diseased conditions of the lachrymal canal, sac, and nasal duct, to the exclusion of all the older methods.

Mr. Bowman's Operation.—In cases of obstruction of the punctum, canaliculus, and nasal duct, resulting in watery eye,

105

accumulation of mucus in the canal, and dryness of the nose, great difficulty used to be experienced in the treatment. To pass a probe along the punctum was extremely difficult, in fact, possible only with a very small one, while the common operation of opening the dilated sac, through the skin, and then passing probes through this artificial opening, was found quite useless from the rapid closure of the wound, unless the treatment was followed up by the insertion and retention of a style in the nasal duct. This was painful, unsightly, often unsuccessful; and even in some cases dangerous, from the amount of irritation, suppuration, and even caries of the nasal bones which is set up.

The principle of Mr. Bowman's most excellent operation is, that the punctum, canaliculus, and nasal duct resemble in many respects the urethral passage, and in cases of stricture require to be treated on the same principle. If, then, it were possible to pass instruments gradually increasing in size through the seat of stricture, it would be gradually dilated. It is, however, in the normal state of parts, impossible to pass any instrument beyond the size of a human hair past the curve which the canaliculus makes on its entrance to the duct, hence the proper dilatation cannot be performed. Again, it is found that the puncta, specially the lower one, are themselves very often to blame, in cases of watery eye, sometimes because they are inverted or everted, more often because, sympathising with the lid, they are turgid, angry, and inflamed, pouting and closed like the orifice of the urethra in a gonorrhœa.

Mr. Bowman found that by slitting up the inferior punctum and canaliculus as far as the caruncula, several advantages were gained:— (1.) The swollen, angry, displaced punctum no longer impeded the entrance of the tears; (2.) and chiefly when the canaliculus was slit up, the curve, or rather angle, which impeded the passage of probes, was done away with, and the nasal duct could be readily and thoroughly dilated.

Operation.—The surgeon stands behind the patient, who is seated, and leans his head on the surgeon's chest. The affected lid is then drawn gently downwards on the cheek, so as to evert and thoroughly expose the lower punctum. Into this the surgeon introduces a fine probe of steel gilt, the first inch of which is very thin, especially at the point, and deeply grooved on one side, exactly like a small (and straight) Syme's stricture director.

Keeping the canal relaxed by relaxing his hold on the lid, the surgeon now gently wriggles the probe along the canaliculus, gradually stretching it as the probe advances, so as to avoid catching of the sides of the canal before the point of the instrument, till he is satisfied that it has fairly entered the nasal duct. He then stretches the eyelid, brings the handle of the probe out over the cheek so as to evert the punctum as much as possible, and then with a fine sharp-pointed knife enters

106

the groove (Fig. ix.), and fairly slits up the punctum and the canal to the full extent. The incision should be as straight as possible, and through the upper wall of the canaliculus. A dexterous turn of the instrument upwards on the forehead will generally enable it to be passed at once fairly into the nose through the nasal duct, the usual rule being observed of passing it downwards and slightly backwards, the handle of the probe passing just over the supraorbital notch.

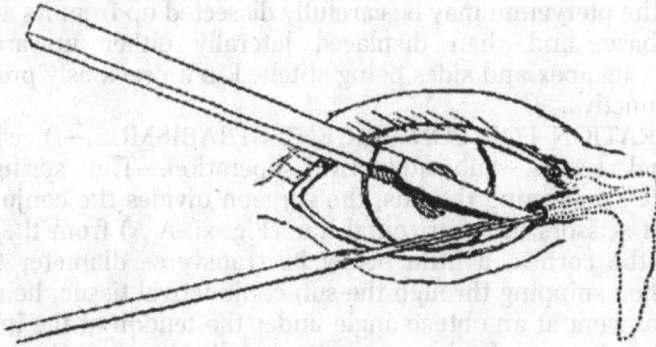

Fig. ix.[83]

For several days after the operation the probe will have to be passed, both to prevent the wound in the canaliculus from healing up, which it is too apt to do, and also to gradually dilate the nasal duct if it has been previously strictured. Probes and directors of various sizes are required; in fact very much the same instruments (in miniature) as are required for the treatment of stricture of the urethra.

Mr. Greenslade has invented a very ingenious little instrument, of which, through his kindness, I am able to show a woodcut (Fig. x.), for slitting up the canaliculus without having to fit the knife in the groove.

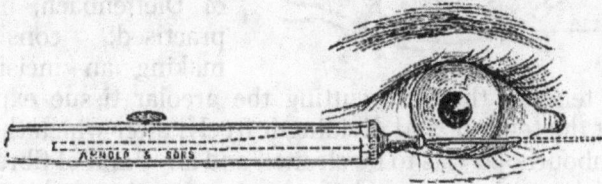

Fig. x.

PTERYGIUM, the reddish fleshy triangular growth, with its base at the inner canthus, and its apex spreading to and often over the

---

[83] Rough diagram of Bowman's operation, showing the grooved director in the punctum, and the knife in the groove just before it slits up the canaliculus.

cornea, requires invariably a small operation for its removal. In most cases it will be found sufficient merely to raise the lax portion over the sclerotic with forceps, and divide it freely, removing a transverse portion. If it has encroached upon the cornea, the portion interfering with vision must be dissected off with great care and removed.

In some cases, however, it has been found that after removal of a large pterygium, a retraction of the caruncle and the semilunar fold is apt to take place, which renders the eyeball unpleasantly prominent. To avoid this the pterygium may be carefully dissected up from its apex to near its base, and then displaced laterally either upwards or downwards, its apex and sides being stitched to a previously prepared site of conjunctiva.

OPERATION FOR CONVERGENT STRABISMUS.—Division of the internal rectus.—Subconjunctival operation.—The spring-wire speculum (C) separating the lids, the surgeon divides the conjunctiva by a pair of scissors in a horizontal line (Fig. xi. A A) from the inner margin of the cornea, a little below its transverse diameter to the caruncle, then snipping through the sub-conjunctival tissue, he passes a blunt hook bent at an obtuse angle under the tendon of the internal rectus, and endeavours by depressing the handle to project the point of the hook at the wound. Then with successive snips of the scissors he divides the tendon on the hook, close to its sclerotic margin. Lest it should not be freely divided, various dips with the hook may be made to catch any stray fibres left untouched; but very great care should be taken not to wound the conjunctiva beyond the first horizontal cut in it. The tendon being divided satisfactorily, the edges of conjunctiva should be replaced, and the eye closed for a few hours.

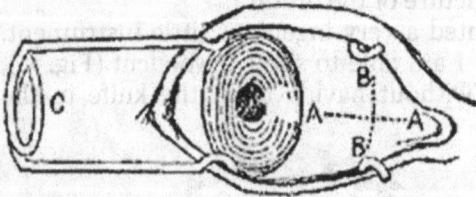

Fig. xi.[84]

The original operation of Dieffenbach, now rarely practised, consisted in making an incision, b b, across the tendon, then, by cutting the areolar tissue exposing the insertion of the tendon, and dividing it freely; after which the sclerotic in the neighbourhood was to be cleaned and any band of fibres divided. There are risks on the one hand of a most unseemly exophthalmos with divergent squint, and on the other of a retraction of the semilunar fold, so that the sub-conjunctival operation is always preferable.

OPERATIONS FOR DIVERGENT SQUINT.—This very serious deformity is often the result of the operation for convergent squint, and

---

[84] Diagram of operations for convergent squint—A A, line of sub-conjunctival incision; B B, line of Dieffenbach's operation; c, wire speculum.

is associated with a fixed, leering, and prominent eye, and frequently with most annoying double vision.

1. In a simple case of primary divergent strabismus (very rare) it is sufficient simply to divide the external rectus in the manner already described for division of the internal.

2. If secondary to an operation for convergent squint, the indication is to restore the cut internal rectus to a position on the sclerotic a little behind its previous one, as the cause of the divergence is found in a complete detachment of the internal rectus. This is attempted in various ways.

(1.) JULES GUÉRIN carefully divided the conjunctiva over it, and sought for the remains of the internal rectus, freeing it from its attachments. He then passed a thread through the sclerotic on the outer side of the globe, and by pulling on it and fixing it across the nose, rotated the eye inwards, in the hope that the remains of the internal rectus would secure a new attachment.

(2.) GRAEFE'S MODIFICATION of this is more certain. Without any minute dissection he merely separated the internal rectus, along with the conjunctiva, and fascia over it, so that it can be pulled forwards, then cut the external rectus, and inverted the eyeball to a sufficient extent by means of a thread passed through the portion of the tendon of the external rectus, which remains attached to the sclerotic. The risk of all these operations, in which both muscles are divided, is protrusion of the eyeball from the removal of muscular tension.

(3.) *Solomon's operation for the radical cure of extreme divergent strabismus*,[85] is at first sight a very curious one. Without going into all the details, the steps are as follows:—

a. A square-shaped flap, with its attached base at the nasal side, is raised, containing the remains of the inner rectus and its adjacent parts.

b. A flap similar in shape and size, but different in the position of its attached base, is made on the other side of the cornea. It is made by dividing the external rectus just behind its tendon, and then reflecting forwards the tendon with its conjunctiva.

c. These two flaps are united over the vertical meridian of the cornea by sutures, three generally being sufficient. This entirely hides the cornea for a time, but eventually shrivels and contracts, and the remnants are to be cut off with scissors three weeks after the operation.

PUNCTURE OF THE CORNEA.—*Paracentesis of the Anterior Chamber.—Tapping of the Aqueous Humour.*—This very simple operation is in many cases extremely useful. In cases of corneal ulcer, the result either of injury or disease, where there is much pain in the bone, and evidence of tension of the globe, it gives great relief, and

---

[85] The Radical Cure of Extreme Divergent Strabismus. J. Vose Solomon, F.R.C.S., 1864.

when repeated at short intervals greatly hastens a cure. Sperino of Turin recommends its frequent use in cases of chronic glaucoma.

Operation.—The surgeon stands behind the patient, who is seated; the lids being fixed, the upper by the surgeon's left hand, and the lower by an assistant, the cornea is punctured a little in front of the sclerotic margin, either with a broad needle, or, what is as good, a well-worn Beer's knife. Care must be taken on entering the knife, on the one hand, not to wound the iris, which is sometimes arched forwards in the cases of commencing glaucoma, and, on the other, fairly to enter the anterior chamber, not merely split up the layers of the cornea. On withdrawing the cataract knife, the aqueous humour gets out by its side, aided by a slight turn of the knife, sometimes with great force, and in much larger quantity than usual. If the operation has been done by a needle, a blunt probe requires to be introduced on the removal of the needle. Once punctured, the remarkable fact is that the same wound suffices for many succeeding tappings, which are effected by pressing the probe into the wound day after day, sometimes several times a day, with great relief to the symptoms. If the probe is to be used for succeeding evacuations, the operator must be careful to remember the exact spot at which the needle or knife was entered. To facilitate remembering it, it is best, when nothing prevents it, to operate always in the same spot. Sperino chooses the horizontal meridian of the cornea at the temporal side, at the junction of the cornea and sclerotic.

CATARACT OPERATIONS.—Here we cannot enter into any discussion of the pathology of cataract and the varieties of it. Enough for our purpose to know that the lens is in some cases hard, in others soft, and that thus in the latter it may be removed piecemeal, and by a small incision, while in the former, removal must be almost entire, and by a larger opening.

In cataract, the lens, which should be transparent, has become opaque, and the object of treatment is to get it out of the line of sight, to prevent it from obstructing, now that it can no longer assist sight.

The operations used for this end may be classed under three heads:—

1. *Operations for the removal of the lens out of the way without its removal from the eye.*—These used to be extensively practised under the name couching, and are of two kinds,—Depression, where the lens is simply pushed down from its place by a needle; Reclination, in which it is shoved backwards (turning on its transverse axis) as well as downwards. These are relics of old surgery, and very rarely practised by any oculists of eminence, as, though easy to perform, and with very flattering immediate results, the risks of chronic inflammation of the whole globe and injury to the retina are very great.

2. *For solution.*—THE NEEDLE OPERATION.—Suitable (among other cases) especially in congenital cataracts in infants, and in cases of diabetic cataract.

110

The principle of this operation is that the lens, once the capsule is freely opened in front and the aqueous humour admitted, is found rapidly to become absorbed and disappear, if the cataract has been a soft one.

Operation.—A needle with a lance-shaped head is to be used. It should be so made that the rounded shaft of the needle is just large enough to play freely in the wound made by the broader point, and yet not so small as to allow the aqueous humour to escape rapidly. The pupil has been dilated, the patient is lying on his back, and the globe is fixed by forceps attached to the conjunctiva of the inner side of the eye, and held by an assistant. The surgeon then enters the needle close to the sclerotic margin of the cornea, carries it fairly on in the anterior chamber, till the centre of the pupil is reached. He then, by bringing forward the handle, projects the point backwards against the anterior capsule, which he freely lacerates with the point and edge in several directions.

In infants, where processes of repair go on very rapidly, the whole lens may be freely broken up. In diabetic cataract, or indeed in all cases of solution, where the patient is adolescent or adult, or the eye at all weak, only a small portion of the lens should be attacked at one sitting.

The needle should then be withdrawn gradually and with great care, that the broad axis of the blade be in exactly the same position in which it entered, i.e. flat and parallel with the iris, lest the iris be wounded, entangled, or prolapsed.

The eye is then to be closed for twenty-four hours; if there is much pain, atropia must be freely used.

Varieties in the Operation.—Some use two needles at once for breaking up the lens. Some surgeons prefer to enter the needle through the sclerotic; this complicates the operation and renders it less certain, as the point of the needle is of course out of sight in its progress between the iris and the lens.

Even in children this operation requires in most cases to be repeated at least once, while in adults it may be required at short intervals for many months.

3. *By Extraction.*—In these operations the lens is at once removed from the eye—

(1.) By linear, or perhaps, more correctly, rectilinear incision. This method is specially suited for cases of soft cataract.

Operation.—A fine spear-shaped needle is very cautiously introduced through the cornea, about a line from its outer margin, and the anterior capsule lacerated, and the lens broken up, great care being taken not to injure the posterior capsule. The pupil must then be kept freely dilated, the wound heals at once, and the aqueous humour reaccumulates.

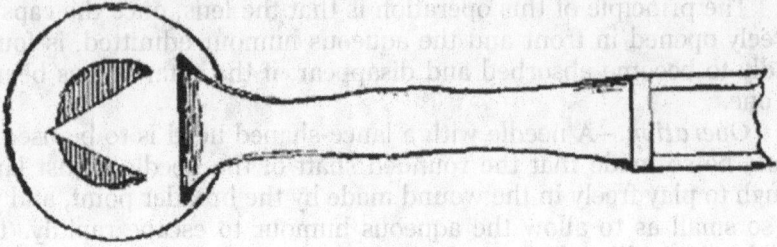

Fig. xii.

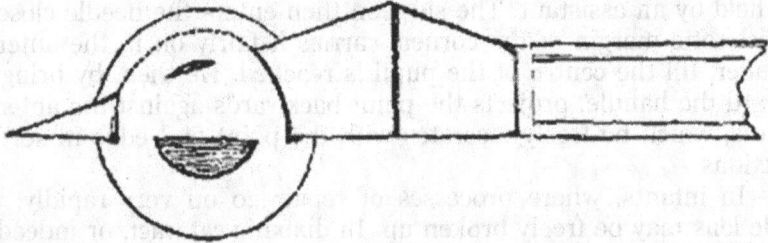

Fig. xiii.

From three to six days after this first operation, a linear incision (Fig. xii.) is made in the outer side of the cornea by a straight stab from a double-edged knife, or rather spear. The size of the incision must vary with the size and consistence of the lens, and can be regulated by the breadth of the knife and the distance to which it is entered. By careful withdrawal of the knife, in many cases a large portion of the soft lens can be removed along with it, and then what remains must be cautiously lifted out by a flat spoon introduced through the wound, and behind the remains of the lens.

Care must be taken lest any of the lens substance remain in the wound; with this precaution the incision generally heals rapidly, and with much less risk of general inflammation of the ball than in the ordinary flap operation of extraction.

EXTRACTION OF SOFT CATARACT BY SUCTION.—Mr. T. P. Teale, of Leeds,[86] has invented an instrument by which the removal of soft cataract is made more easy, through a linear incision by suction, applied through the medium of a hollow curette furnished with an india-rubber tube and mouth-piece.

The curette is of the usual size, but is roofed in (instead of being merely grooved) to within one line of its extremity, thus forming a tube flattened above, but terminating in a small cup. This is screwed into an ordinary straight handle, which is hollow for a short distance, far enough to join with a second tube fixed

---

[86] Ophthalmic Hospital Reports, vol. iv. part ii. p. 197.

at right angles to the handle, and into which the india-rubber pipe and mouth-piece, through which suction is to be made, is attached. In many cases it seems to serve its purpose extremely well.

Certain points require attention:—1. That the puncture to admit the curette is large enough; 2. That its end be sufficiently rounded; 3. Its open end must be held in the area of the pupil, and not allowed to pass behind the iris, else there is great risk of the iris being drawn in. Among other advantages claimed by its inventor, the chief seems to be a more thorough removal of the lens than by the ordinary means, and consequently less risk of opaque deposit in the posterior capsule.

(2.) EXTRACTION BY FLAP.—When properly performed in a suitable subject, and when free from accident, this operation is one of the most thoroughly beautiful and satisfactory in the whole domain of surgery; but it is difficult, and liable to many risks which neither skill nor caution can completely guard against.

It is required in many cases of hard cataract, which are amenable neither to solution nor linear extraction.

Operation must be considered in various stages:—

a. To make a flap of cornea large enough to permit of the removal of the entire lens without pressure or bruising. To make it of cornea only, to prevent the escape of the vitreous, and to avoid injury of the iris.

The great difficulty in making the required section of the cornea is, that we are debarred from using scissors or any ordinary knife or scalpel in making it, for this reason, that the sawing movements required in all ordinary cutting are inadmissible here, as any withdrawal of the blade, however slight, would permit evacuation of the aqueous humour, and at once be followed by prolapse of the iris before the knife. Hence we are compelled to make the requisite flap by one steady push of a knife, which, too, must be of such a shape as in its entrance constantly to fill up the wound it makes. Very various shapes and sizes of knives have been proposed, the one called Beer's knife being the sort of model or common parent from which all the others are derived. It is triangular in shape, with a straight back, about 12-10ths of an inch in length, and 4-10ths broad at the base of the blade, tapering at a straight edge from its base to its point, and also diminishing in thickness to the point.

Considerable difference of opinion exists as to the relative merits of an upper or lower section of the cornea. The general view at present seems to be that an upper section is to be preferred; but in cases where the surgeon is not ambidexterous, it is better that he should make the section which lies easiest to his hand than attempt an upper section in a less favourable position.

The patient should be placed flat on his back, the lids should be

113

gently opened, the upper one by the surgeon, the lower one by his assistant, who is to press the lid downwards against the malar bone without exercising any pressure on the ball. The eye should be still further steadied by the conjunctiva and subjacent cellular tissue on the inner side being seized by a pair of catch-forceps, still with no downward pressure on the ball. The point of the knife must then be introduced about a line from the outer sclerotic margin of the transverse diameter of the cornea (Fig. xiii.), the blade being held parallel with the fibres of the iris, pushed steadily across the anterior chamber, and protruded as nearly as possible at the corresponding spot at the inner side of the cornea. The aqueous humour should not escape till the section is completed. If it does, the iris is almost certainly projected forwards and entangled in the blade of the knife, a most annoying accident, and one which is not easily remedied. The books tell us of various manœuvres by pressure or otherwise, by which the iris may be pushed back. Practically, however, if it has once occurred it is not easily saved from being cut. If a small portion only is involved, it is not of much consequence; if a large portion be in danger, it is sometimes necessary to withdraw the knife before the section is completed, and finish it with a probe-pointed, curved bistoury.

If, however, the flap is safely finished, the lids should be gently allowed to close for a few seconds.

On opening them again the surgeon must decide whether the corneal flap is sufficiently large to allow the lens to come out without force; if not, he must enlarge it either by the narrow probe-pointed "secondary knife" or by a pair of sharp scissors. Occasionally the lens, and even a little vitreous humour, may escape at once on the section being completed, but this is not to be desired.

b. *Laceration of the Capsule of the Lens.*—This is performed by insinuating a sharp curved needle under the corneal flap, avoiding the iris, and then tearing up the anterior capsule through the dilated pupil, the chief point to be attended to being that the capsule be lacerated in its entire length.

c. *Removal of the Lens.*—This must be done with the most extreme caution and gentleness, lest the vitreous humour be also evacuated. The surgeon's object is to tilt the lens so as to turn it slightly on its transverse axis, and cause the edge nearest the section to rise out of the capsule and appear at the wound. This is best done by gentle pressure at the required spot by the back of the needle, or by a common probe. When the lens begins to protrude the pressure must be very gentle, lest it be forced out suddenly and the vitreous follow it.

Soft portions of the lens are apt to remain adherent to the wound in the cornea. These must be removed by scoop or probe.

Varieties in the method of Flap Extraction.—Jacobsen of Königsberg in every case gives chloroform. He always makes his flap in the boundary line of the cornea and the sclerotic, through a vascular

114

structure, and he believes that union is on this account more rapid, and after extraction removes that portion of the iris which appears to have been most exposed to bruising during the exit of the lens.

The operation of extraction may in many cases be either preceded or followed by iridectomy, as proposed by Mooren, Von Graefe, and others. The following operation seems to diminish the risks to a very great extent:—

Professor Von Graefe's Operation.—The lids are separated by a speculum, and the eyeball is drawn down by forceps placed immediately below the cornea. The point of a small knife, of which the edge is directed upwards, is inserted at a point fully half a line from the margin of the cornea near its upper part, so as to enter the anterior chamber as peripherally as possible. The point should not be directed at first towards the spot for counterpuncture; nor till the knife has advanced fully three and a half lines within the visible portion of the anterior chamber, should the handle be lowered and the point directed so as to make a symmetrical counterpuncture, which will give the external wound a length of four and a half or five lines. As soon as the resistance to the point is felt to be overcome, showing that the counterpuncture is effected, the knife must at once be turned forward, so that its back is directed almost to the centre of the ideal sphere of the cornea, whether the conjunctiva is transfixed or not, and the scleral border is divided by boldly pushing the knife onwards and again drawing it backwards. This portion of the operation is concluded by the formation of a conjunctival flap a line and a half or two lines in length. A section thus made is almost perpendicular to the cornea, a circumstance much facilitating the passage of the lens, and the line of incision is nearly straight, so that the wound does not gape. The iris should be excised to the very end of the wound, and the capsule most freely opened by a V-shaped laceration. Any lens, even the hardest, may then be removed without the introduction of an instrument into the eye, but Von Graefe's experience shows it to be advisable to assist the evacuation by the hook in about one case in eight. In a certain number of cases the lens will escape without difficulty when the operator presses on the posterior lip of the wound, especially when the back of the spoon is made to glide along the sclera; should this not occur, Von Graefe uses a peculiar blunt hook, or occasionally, though rarely, a spoon. A compressing bandage is applied, and replaced at intervals.[87]

We are recommended to perform it in two sets of cases:—
1. Those in which the eye is known to be unhealthy and liable to

---

[87] Biennial Retrospect for 1865-66. Syd. Soc. pp. 363-4. For a thorough discussion of the merits of this operation, see papers by Von Graefe in Brit. Med. Jour. for 1867, vol. i. pp. 379, 446, 499, 657, 765.

inflammations, specially of iris, retina, or choroid. In cases where the patient has already lost an eye, Von Graefe thinks iridectomy should always precede extraction. In the above, then, it is a precautionary measure, and, if convenient, should be performed three, four, or even six weeks before the extraction.

2. It is recommended to be performed at the same time as extraction in all cases in which the operation has presented any special difficulties, or has not gone smoothly, e.g. in cases where the lens has required much force to expel it, either from the flap of cornea being too small, or from adhesions between the lens and capsule; or, again, in cases in which there is a tendency to prolapse of the iris, in which any of the cortical substance has been necessarily left behind, or in which old adhesions had existed between the iris and capsule, or between the cornea and iris.

OPERATIONS FOR ARTIFICIAL PUPIL.—The cases are by no means unfrequent in which it is necessary to remove or destroy a portion of the iris to admit light to the retina. In cases of excessive prolapse of the iris after extraction of the lens, where the iris has formed adhesions to the wound, and still more frequently in cases where central opacities of the cornea have fairly occluded the natural pupil, the only chance for vision is to enlarge the old one, or make a new pupil by removal of the iris.

Very various operations have been proposed, and exceedingly numerous and complicated instruments invented for this purpose. We can notice here only one or two of the most approved procedures:—

1. Incision is the simplest.

This is practicable and effectual only in cases where the iris is so far healthy as still to retain its contractile power, and so far free from adhesions as to be able to make use of it. The best example of such a case is that of a cataract, in which after extraction a prolapse of the iris has occurred to such an extent as to obliterate the pupil, and where, at the same time, the only adhesions are to the wound, none to the cornea.

Operation.—A double-edged needle is introduced through the cornea near its margin; on arriving at the place where the pupil ought to be, one edge is drawn against the iris, and divides it transversely, if possible, without injuring the lens; the fibres of the iris start back, contract, so that a sufficiently large central pupil may be obtained.

2. Excision.—In the far more frequent cases in which there exist adhesions between iris and cornea, or iris and anterior capsule, incision is not sufficient, and it is necessary to excise a portion of the iris.

The simplest and safest operation is the following:—

The patient recumbent, and the lids held apart by a speculum, the eyeball should be steadied by the forceps of an assistant. A broad cutting needle should then be introduced at the lower or outer edge of the corneal margin. This must be very gently withdrawn so as to retain as much aqueous humour as possible. Into the wound thus made the surgeon must introduce the blunt hook (known as Tyrrell's) at first with its point forwards, then, on arriving opposite the edge of the pupil, which it is intended to enlarge or replace, with its point turned backwards, so as to hook over the edge of the iris and thus drag on it. Once the hook has fairly got hold, it must again be rotated forwards, and withdrawn in the same direction as it was put in. The iris thus pulled out of the wound is to be cut off with a pair of fine scissors, so as to remove a sufficient amount to make a new pupil of the required size.

But in those cases in which the whole or greater part of the pupillary margin is adherent, the blunt hook will not do, because there exists no edge round which to hook it. One of two plans is generally chosen to remedy this:—

(1.) A free incision made with a double-edged needle; through this a pair of canula forceps is introduced, with which a portion of iris is seized and dragged to the external wound; it can then either be cut off or tied (see Iridesis); or,

(2.) A previous attempt may be made to free a portion to form an edge to catch hold of, either by incision or by Corelysis (q.v.).

IRIDESIS.—Critchett's Operation of Ligature.[88]—Patient being put under chloroform, the ball is fixed by the wire speculum, and also by a fold of conjunctiva being seized by forceps. An opening is then made with a broad needle through the margin of the cornea, close to the sclerotic, just large enough to admit the canula forceps, with which a small portion of iris close to its ciliary attachment is seized and drawn out; a piece of fine floss silk, previously tied in a small loop round the canula forceps, is slipped down and carefully tightened round the prolapsed portion. This speedily shrinks, and the loop may generally be removed about the second day. The chief advantage claimed for this method is the ease with which the size of the new pupil can be regulated. It is also suitable in cases of conical cornea, where it is wished to change the form of the pupil into a narrow slit.

N.B.—The ends of the ligature must be left sufficiently long to avoid any risk of their being drawn out of sight into the substance of the cornea, or even into the ball, by retraction of the fibres of the iris.

CORELYSIS.—*Freeing of the Pupil.*—An operative procedure for separating posterior adhesions of the iris to the lens. In it the surgeon hopes to act, not on the iris, as in the operations for artificial pupil, but only on the bands of false membrane which distort the pupil.

The operation is briefly as follows:—The eye being firmly held by a wire speculum, and forceps pinching up the conjunctiva, a broad needle is passed rapidly through the cornea at a point which may give easy access to the adhesion to be torn through. This point is generally

---

[88] Ophthalmic Hospital Reports, vol. i. p. 224.

at the opposite margin of the irregular pupil, so that the needle may pass through the cornea in front of the one side of the iris, then through the orifice of the pupil, so as to reach the back of the other side. The needle is withdrawn gradually, so as to lose as little of the aqueous humour as possible, and then the spatula hook, called after the inventor of the operation, Mr. Streatfeild, is introduced. It is used first as a spatula, that is, with its blunt, though polished edge, to separate the adhesions, and if this is unsuccessful, as a hook (Fig. xiv.), so as to catch and tear them. In cases which resist the instrument used in both of these ways, Mr. Streatfeild has used very fine canula-scissors to cut the adhesions.[89] Such a further complication of the operation practically alters its character into an operation for artificial pupil, q.v.

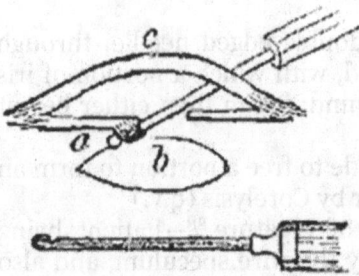

Fig. xiv.[90]

IRIDECTOMY.—In cases of acute glaucoma, irido-choroiditis, and all deep inflammations of the eye in which the ocular tension is increased, also in certain cases of flap extraction already alluded to, the operation of iridectomy as originally proposed by Von Graefe will be found of use.

Operation.—The patient recumbent, and the eye absolutely fixed by speculum and forceps, a linear incision, varying in length from one-sixth to one-fourth of an inch, is made just at the margin of the cornea. The point of election is the upper pole of the cornea. The lens must not be wounded. The best instrument for making the section is an ordinary linear extraction knife, bent at an angle to admit of its being introduced from above. The iris will protrude through the wound, or, if adherent, must be drawn out by forceps, and then is to be cut off with scissors. The operation is rarely successful, unless a third, or at least a fourth, of the iris be removed.

EXCISION OF A STAPHYLOMATOUS CORNEA.—There are certain cases in which the whole or greater part of the cornea bulges forward in a great blue projecting tumour. It is very ugly as it protrudes between the lids and prevents their closure; besides this, from its exposure it frequently inflames, even ulcerates, and has a most injurious effect on the other eye. In the cases suitable for operation vision is completely gone, without hope of its restoration by any operative procedure.

---

[89] Streatfeild on Corelysis. Ophthalmic Hospital Reports, vol. ii. p. 309.
[90] a iris; b lens; c cornea. The hook is seen applied to the adhesion between lens and iris.

The best thing for the patient is to have just enough of the staphyloma removed to enable the remains of the eyeball to form a good stump for an artificial eye. Various means have been suggested for doing this, varying in extent and severity from a mere shaving off the apex of the staphyloma to excision of the whole eyeball.

By far the best method of operating is the one proposed and practised by Mr. Critchett.

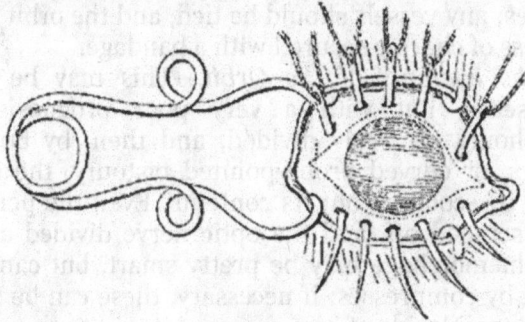

Fig. xv.[91]

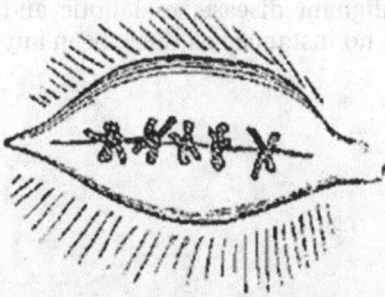

Fig. xvi.[92]

The object of it is to remove an elliptical portion of the front of the staphyloma, or the whole staphyloma, when it is possible, and at the same time to prevent as far as possible the escape of the vitreous.

Operation.—Three, four, or five small curved needles armed with thread are passed through the staphyloma from above downwards, being each entered a little above the line of the intended upper incision, and brought out a little below the line of the intended lower one (Fig. xv.)

To remove the included elliptical portion, Mr. Critchett pierces the sclerotic with a Beer's knife, just in front of the tendinous insertion of the external rectus. Through this incision a pair of probe-pointed scissors is introduced, and the piece cut just within the points of the needles. On the removal, the needles, which have retained the vitreous by their pressure, are drawn through and the threads cautiously tied.

Union by first intention very often occurs, and an excellent stump is left with a narrow depressed transverse cicatrix[93] (Fig. xvi.)

---

[91] The staphyloma with the needles inserted, the lids held asunder by a spring speculum. The elliptical dotted line shows the amount to be removed; the vertical one, the position of the preliminary incision with the Beer's knife.
[92] Resulting stump after the stitches are inserted.

119

EXTIRPATION OF THE EYEBALL.—1. *Of the Eyeball only.*—A circular incision should be made with curved scissors through the conjunctiva, a little beyond the corneal margin, then, beginning with the external rectus, muscle after muscle should be raised with the forceps, and divided, after which the optic nerve is cut through with the scissors. A slight preliminary extension outwards of the optic commissure will facilitate the dissection, and must be secured with metallic sutures; any vessels should be tied, and the orbit filled up with a light compress of charpie secured with a bandage.

2. *Of the contents of the Orbit.*—This may be required for malignant disease, but with a very poor prognosis. The optic commissure should be freely divided, and then, by bold strokes of curved scissors, or curved probe-pointed bistoury, the orbit may be fairly emptied by scooping out its contents. Even the periosteum may require to be scraped off, and the optic nerve divided as far back as possible. The hæmorrhage may be pretty smart, but can generally be easily checked by compresses; if necessary, these can be soaked in the solution of the perchloride of iron.

The author has done this operation many times, in cases extensive and of old standing, for malignant disease, melanotic and encephaloid. All have recovered, and in no instance has there been any trouble in stopping the bleeding.

93 Ophthalmic Hospital Reports, vol. iv. part 1.

CHAPTER VI

OPERATIONS ON THE NOSE AND LIPS

RHINOPLASTIC OPERATIONS.—The operations for the restoration or repair of lost or mutilated noses are so various, and the minuteness of detail necessary for full description of them so great, that a complete account in a manual such as this is impossible; a brief notice of some of the most important varieties of the operation is all that can be given.

Principles.—1. It is necessary in every case that a suitable edge be prepared on which to fix the flap of skin, however obtained. To be suitable, this edge, should be (a) made in healthy skin, not in old or weak cicatrices; hence no trace of the original disease should be left; (b) it should be made thoroughly raw, by the removal of an appreciable amount of its edge; it should be pared, not merely scraped.

2. It is useless to attempt to restore a nose unless the patient is in good general health, well nourished, and perfectly free from all remains of disease in the nose or its neighbourhood. The flaps which are to form the new nose may be obtained either from (1.) the cheeks; (2.) the forehead; (3.) a distant part either of the patient or of another person.

(1.) *From the Cheeks.*—When the cheeks are healthy, and specially if they are tolerably full and lax, the flaps from the cheeks produce much the most satisfactory result. As performed by Mr. Syme, the operation consists in the shaping of two equal flaps (a, a) from the skin of the cheek at each side, having the attachment above. A site for each flap is formed by the careful paring away of the whole thickness of the edge of the cavity of the lost organ (see Fig. xvii.)

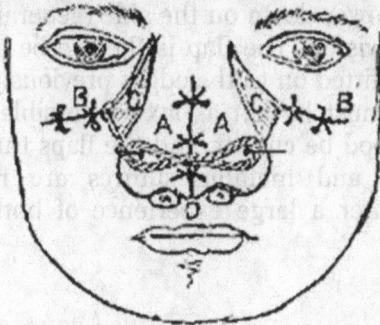

Fig. xvii.[94]

---

[94] Operation for formation of a new nose from the cheeks; a a, flaps approximated in middle line; B B, outer part of bed of flaps stitched up; C C, triangle at each side left to granulate.

121

The flaps are then raised from their attachments to the upper jaw-bone, and approximated in the middle line by several points of metallic suture and the outer edges stitched to the raw surface on each side at a proper distance from the nasal orifice. If any septum remains of the old nose, it may be made very useful as a fixed point, a straight needle being thrust through one flap close to its outer lower edge, then through the septum, and out at a corresponding point of the other flap. The edges of the wound left in the cheek at each side can generally be, to a certain extent, approximated by silver stitches (b, b) and the triangular portion (c, c), which is necessarily left to heal by granulation, proves an advantage, as by its depression it enhances the apparent height and prominence of the new organ. The cavity should be very gently distended with lint, and may be supported by the blades of a small pair of forceps, applied so as to embrace the nose.

(2.) *From the Forehead.*—The Indian operation may be used as a last resource, in cases where, from disease, the cheeks also have suffered, and are not to be trusted to for flaps.

Operation.—1. It should be decided as to the shape and size of the portion of skin necessary, by fitting on pieces of soft leather or moulding wax. To allow for shrinking, the flap should be made at least one-third larger than is at first apparently necessary. The exact boundaries of the flap to be raised should then be marked out on the forehead by lightly pencilling it with nitrate of silver, the mark from which is not effaced by blood, as is sure to be the case with an ink line. Various shapes have been proposed for the flap varying in length of neck, in the shape of the angles, and especially in the arrangements made for the formation of a columna. Some (as Liston) prefer afterwards to provide for the columns separately, by a flap raised from the upper lip in a subsequent operation. The flap is then to be raised from the forehead, care being taken not to injure the periosteum. The incision is to be carried lower down on the side (generally the left), to which the flap is to be twisted. The flap is then to be brought round (Fig. xviii.) and carefully fitted on to the edges previously prepared for its reception. The neck must be left as lax as possible, lest by tight twisting the supply of blood be cut off, and the flaps thus deprived of nourishment. Both silk and metallic sutures are recommended. Hamilton of Dublin,[95] after a large experience of both, prefers the former.

---

[95] The Restoration of a Lost Nose by Operation, p. 57; an excellent monograph on the subject.

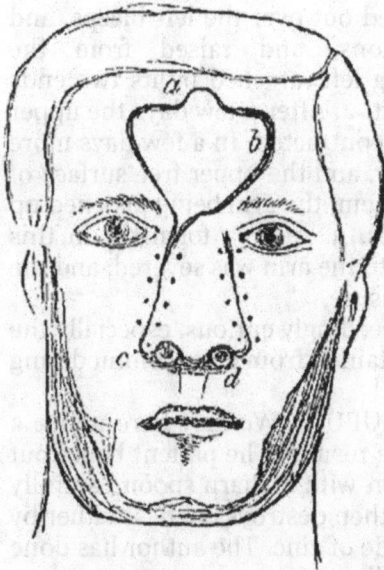

Fig. xviii.[96]

There are various risks; sloughing of the whole flap at once, shrinking of it after weeks or even months; certain inevitable drawbacks, as the cicatrix on the forehead, the very various and ludicrous changes of colour to which the new organ is subject,—these cannot be remedied by further operation. Two points generally require a second use of the knife a few weeks after:—(1.) The neck of the flap is sure to be redundant and prominent, but can be pared. (2.) The columna almost always requires improving, and, in Liston's method, to be made. He pared the inner surface of the apex of the nose, and then raised a central flap of the lip in the middle line, about a quarter of an inch broad, and extending from the remains of the old septum to the free border, raising it from the gum, and stitched the free end of it to the prepared apex, bringing together the two divided portions of the lip by ordinary harelip sutures. Tho columna, if redundant, could be shaved down, and it was found that the mucous surface very quickly became like skin on exposure.

For other points with regard to the operation, reference may be made to the works of Liston and Skey, and Hamilton's monograph, referred to above.

Note.—The tongue and groove suture proposed by Professor Pancoast, and recommended by Professor Gross, is said to be specially suitable for such plastic operations. It is very complicated, as it requires one edge to be bevelled to a wedge shape, the other being grooved to include the wedge, thus opposing four raw surfaces, which are retained in contact by being transfixed by fine silk sutures.

(3.) There are certain cases in which neither cheeks nor forehead are available for flaps, and yet the patients press very much for some operation. If they have patience and determination, the Taliacotian or Italian operation may be attempted.

Without going into detail, the principle of it is as follows:—1. A

---

[96] Operation for formation of a new nose from the forehead:—a, prominence of flap which is to be used as septum; b, left-hand corner of flap, which is twisted and fastened at c; d, one of the tubes or quills over which the nose is moulded.—(Modified from Bernard and Huette.)

piece of skin of suitable size was marked out over the left biceps, and defined by two longitudinal incisions, and raised from the subcutaneous cellular tissue, thus being left attached by its two ends only; a piece of linen was pulled below it. 2. After a few days the upper end was also divided, and the flap thus contracted. In a few days more the sides of the old nose were made raw, and the upper free surface of the flap also made raw and stitched to them, the arm being fastened up by a most elaborate series of bandages. 3. After a fortnight in this position, the last attachment of the flap to the arm was severed, and the new nose could then be modelled at pleasure.

The literature of the subject is exceedingly curious, especially the cases in which the new material was obtained from an accommodating friend or servant.

OPERATIVE TREATMENT OF LUPUS.—We may here notice a mode of treatment which has admirable results. The patient being put deeply under an anæsthetic, the surgeon with a sharp spoon carefully pares away all the diseased tissues, and then destroys the base either by nitric acid or a strong solution of chloride of zinc. The author has done this in a great number of cases with excellent effect.

NASAL POLYPI, *Removal of.*—Of these there are different kinds.

1. ORDINARY MUCOUS POLYPI.—These grow from the spongy bones, generally the superior one, are non-malignant in their character, soft and vascular, often fill up the whole of both nasal cavities, and frequently hang down behind into the pharynx. The practical point to remember is that, however large and numerous they may be, they invariably have their origin from a comparatively limited spot, the edge of the spongy bone, and always hang from a narrow neck. Hence the treatment is easy and satisfactory, if the neck be attacked, and not the body of the tumour.

Slightly curved, narrow-bladed forceps should be passed along by the side of the superior spongy bone, with their blades open, till the neck of the polypus is seized. Holding it firmly, the forceps should then be slowly twisted round till the neck is destroyed and the polypus detached. This should be repeated till the patient can blow freely through both nostrils. If attempts are made to seize the body of the polypus, it will break down under the forceps, bleed, and give much trouble.

2. THE FIBROUS POLYPUS.—This form is fortunately much more rare than the other. It is almost invariably single, is attached to the posterior margin of the nares by a narrow but very strong root, is extremely firm in consistence, may grow to a large size so as to obstruct both nostrils, generally gives rise to severe and frequent hæmorrhages. The hæmorrhage during any attempt to remove it is generally of the most severe character, but ceases immediately on its complete detachment.

We owe nearly all that we do know about the treatment of this form of polypus to Mr. Syme. His method is—By the ordinary polypus forceps described already, he seized the tumour through the nostril, and then with the fore and middle fingers of the left hand introduced behind the soft palate, he attacked the point of attachment, and by his nails, aided by the forceps, detached it from its narrow base.[97]

3. MALIGNANT POLYPI should not be meddled with unless it is absolutely certain that the whole of the bone from which they grow can be removed also. This is very rarely the case. (See Excision of Superior Maxilla.)

OPERATIONS ON THE LIPS.—1. Epithelial cancers of the lower lip are very frequent, and require removal.

Fig.xix.[98]

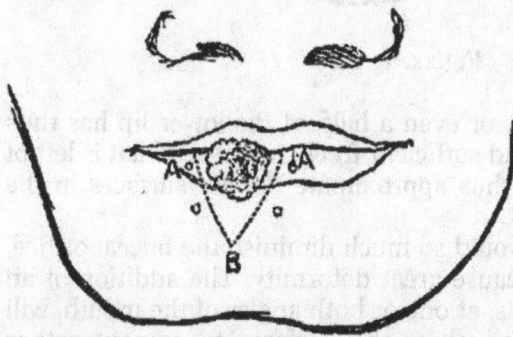

If the tumour or ulcer is small, and involves a considerable thickness of the lip, it is most easily removed by a V-shaped incision (Fig. xix. A B A). Its shape permits the most accurate apposition of the cut surfaces; and if the lips are full and the tumour small, very slight trace of the operation will remain.

Again, if the tumour be more extensive, involving a large portion of the prolabium, and yet not extending deeply into the substance of the lip, it may be very easily removed by a pair of curved scissors, applied in the direction shown in the diagram (Fig. xx. A B). The skin must then be stitched to the mucous membrane by numerous points of interrupted suture.

But if the tumour be at once extensive and deep, mere removal is not sufficient, but some provision must be made for supplying the blank left by the operation.

[97] Syme's Observations in Clinical Surgery, p. 132.
[98] Diagram of V-shaped incision; A B A, dots showing points for sutures.

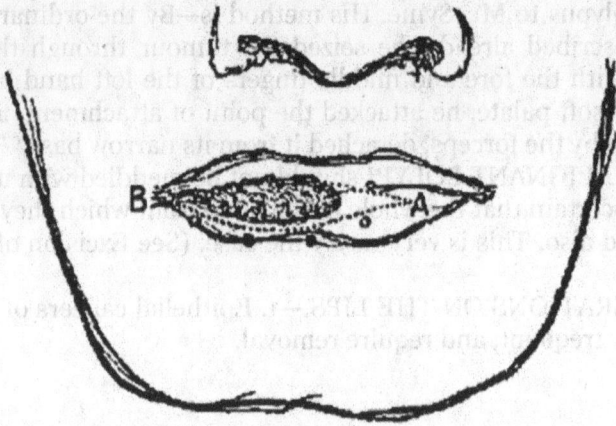

Fig.xx.[99]

In cases where a third, or even a half, of the lower lip has thus been removed, it may be found sufficient freely to dissect what is left of the lip from the gums, and thus approximate the cut surfaces in the middle line.

This alone, however, would so much diminish the buccal orifice, and twist its corners, as to cause great deformity. The addition of an incision horizontally outwards, at one or both angles of the mouth, will do away with such risk, and allow the surfaces to come together without puckering; while by stitching the skin and mucous membrane together in the course of these horizontal incisions, we can increase the size of the buccal orifice almost ad libitum.

Lastly, when the lower lip has been entirely removed, it is still possible to supply its place in the following manner, which was devised by Mr. Syme: The tumour being fairly isolated by a V-shaped incision (Fig. xxi.) C A C including the whole thickness of the lip, each of the incisions should be prolonged downwards and outwards, as shown by the dotted lines A D, A D. The flaps thus marked out must be separated from the bone, brought upwards, and approximated in the middle line. Possibly it may be necessary still further to enlarge the buccal orifice by short lateral incisions, C C. Whether these are required or not, silk stitches are to be introduced to unite the skin and mucous membrane along the lines a c. The gap left between D B D must be left to granulate, but in most cases may be very much diminished in size by additional sutures at its outer corners, near d. The granulating surface E E very rapidly heals up, leaving a dimple on each side, which rather improves the appearance, by adding to the prominence of the chin, b.

---

[99] Diagram of incision for scooping out a shallow tumour by scissors.

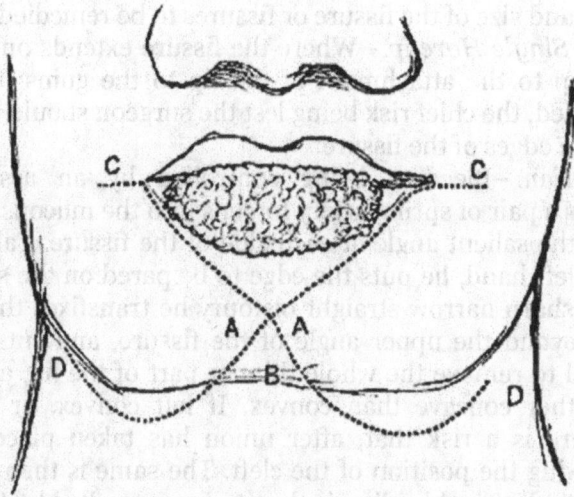

Fig. xxi.[100]

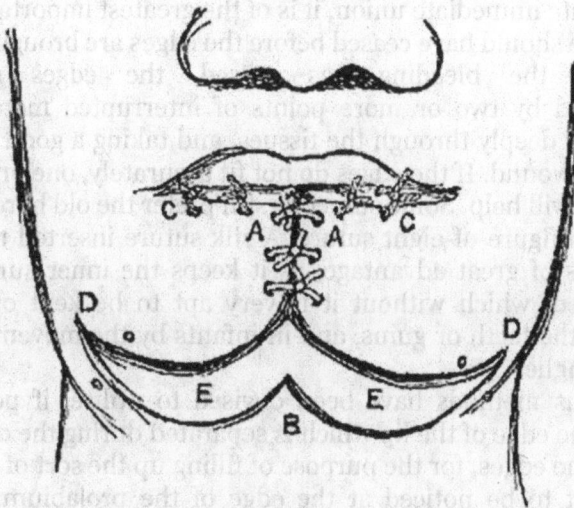

Fig. xxii.[101]

The Operations for Harelip, though all conducted on the same general principles, vary considerably in extent required according to

---

[100] Diagram of incisions:—C A C, outline of incision for removal; C A D, outline of flap on each side; b, prominence of chin; C C, dotted lines, showing incisions to enlarge mouth, if required.

[101] Diagram of flaps in position:—A A, corners of flaps brought up and approximated by silver sutures; C C, new lip got by lateral incisions, skin and mucous membrane being united by silk threads; E E, gap left to granulate.

127

the position and size of the fissure or fissures to be remedied.

1. *For Single Harelip.*—Where the fissure extends only from the prolabium up to the attachment of the lip to the gums: this is very easily remedied, the chief risk being lest the surgeon should not remove enough of the edges of the fissure.

Operation.—Bleeding being controlled by an assistant, the surgeon fixes a pair of spring artery forceps into the mucous membrane and skin at the salient angle at each side of the fissure. Taking one of these in his left hand, he puts the edge to be pared on the stretch, and then with a sharp narrow straight bistoury he transfixes the lip at the point just beyond the upper angle of the fissure, and cuts outwards, being careful to remove the whole thinner part of the lip, and to leave the edge rather concave than convex. If left convex, or even quite straight, there is a risk that, after union has taken place, an angle remain showing the position of the cleft. The same is then to be done on the other side. The bleeding is then to be controlled by twisting the larger vessels, and if oozing still continues from the smaller ones, a pad of lint should be placed in the wound, and a few minutes' delay given, as, to facilitate immediate union, it is of the greatest importance that all hæmorrhage should have ceased before the edges are brought together.

When the bleeding has ceased, the edges should be approximated by two or more points of interrupted metallic suture inserted very deeply through the tissues, and taking a good hold of the edges of the wound. If the edges do not fit accurately, one or two horse-hair sutures will help. Some surgeons still prefer the old harelip needles secured by a figure-of-eight suture. A silk suture inserted through the prolabium is of great advantage, as it keeps the inner surface of the wound closed, which without it is very apt to be kept open by the pressure of the teeth or gums, and in infants by the movements of the tip of the tongue.

Various methods have been devised to utilise, if possible, the portion of the edge of the lip which is separated during the operation of refreshing the edges, for the purpose of filling up the sort of cleft or gap which is apt to be noticed at the edge of the prolabium. The most ingenious and simplest of these is that proposed by M. Nelaton, for use in cases where the fissure does not extend so far up as the nose. It consists in leaving the two portions which are pared off (Fig. xxiii.) the sides of the cleft attached to each other as well as to the free edge of the lip, then pulling them down, so as to bring their bleeding surfaces into apposition, and make a diamond-shaped wound instead of a triangular cleft (Fig. xxiv.) When brought together by sutures a projection is left at the edge of the lip; this, in most cases, disappears; if it does not, it can easily be pared down.

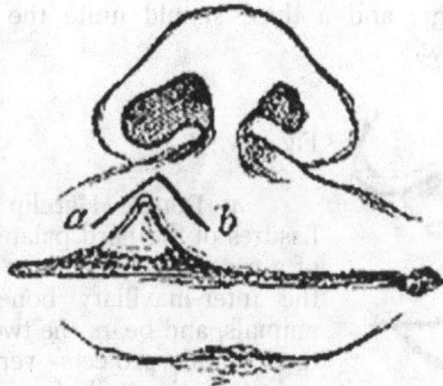

Fig.xxiii.

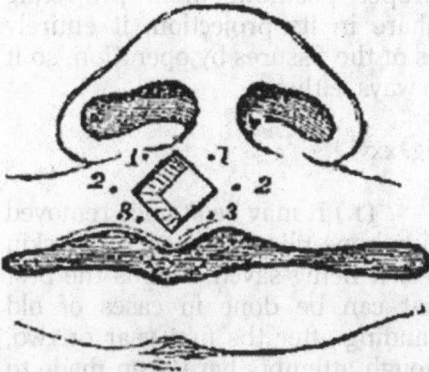

Fig.xxiv.[102]

2. When the fissure, though single, extends upwards into the nose, the operation is more difficult, and the result frequently less satisfactory. The first thing to be done is to separate the lips from the gums, so as to make them more freely mobile. The whole edges of the cleft require refreshing.

3. *Double Harelip*, without bony deformity, and where the intervening portion of the skin is vertical, does not project, and can be made useful for the new lip. Such cases are not very common, but when they do occur the question arises, How are they to be managed—in two separate operations or at once? I believe, in every case, at once. The central wedge-shaped portion is not large enough to extend downwards as far as the prolabium, but still should not be removed altogether, as it may be of great use, especially in bearing the columna nasi, and allowing its full development. The edges should be pared in the same way, and to the same extent as in single harelip, with the addition that the intervening portion should have its edges completely removed, and be left in the form of a wedge, with its apex downwards. The highest suture should be passed through first one side, then the base of the wedge, and then the other side; the second one through both, and the

[102] Fig. xxiv. shows the diamond-shaped wound before the sutures are applied.

129

apex of the wedge; and a third should unite the prolabium, not including the wedge.

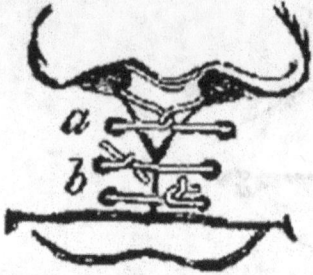

Fig. xxv.[103]

4. Double Harelip combined with fissures of the hard palate, and projection of a central bone. This is the analogue of the inter-maxillary bone in the lower animals, and bears the two middle incisor teeth, and projects very variously in different cases. In some it projects horizontally forwards in the most hideous manner, in others it lies at an angle more or less oblique; in very few does it maintain its proper position; when projecting forwards, and as the teeth also share in its projection, it entirely prevents approximation of the edges of the fissures by operation, so it must first be dealt with in one of two ways, either—

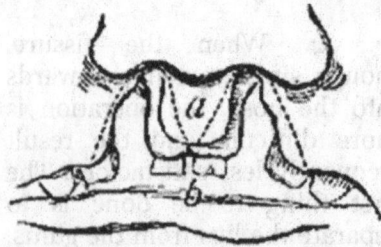

Fig. xxvi.[104]

(1.) It may be at once removed with bone-pliers, the piece of skin over it being saved. This is the best that can be done in cases of old standing after the first year or two, though attempts have been made to break the neck of the projecting portion, and thus permit of its being shoved back.

(2.) By gradual pressure by a spring truss, strapping, or a bandage, it may be forced back. This is possible only in cases where the deformity has been comparatively slight, and the patient has been seen early. The edges must then be pared and approximated as directed above.

One or two points about the operation for harelip require a special notice:—

1. *When to operate.*—Great differences in opinion exist. Some say not before two or three years, others within two or three days, or even hours, after birth.

---

[103] Diagram of operation for double harelip:—a, stitch through both sides and wedge-shaped portion, which also aids the septum; b, other stitches approximating edges.

[104] Diagram of double harelip, with projecting bone:—a, central piece of lip, dotted lines showing incision; b, projecting bone bearing teeth, which are generally small and stunted.

Probably the safest time is not much earlier than the second month in very strong children, the fifth in weakly ones, up to the commencement of the first dentition; and when once dentition has commenced it is not so safe to operate till it is over.

Prior to dentition the operation is attended with rather more risk, but again, if delayed, there is great risk that the teeth do not come in properly.

2. With regard to the most delicate part of the operation, the management of the prolabium.—Some are satisfied, and I believe rightly, with careful apposition by a silk suture after a sufficient amount of the edges has been removed; others have proposed various plans to obviate any risk of an angle remaining.

Malgaigne proposes to retain a small portion of the parings of the edge to make small flap at each side; Lloyd a single one from the long half of the lip, and brings it up under the opposite one, securing it with a stitch.

CHAPTER VII

OPERATIONS ON THE JAWS

1. EXCISION OF THE UPPER JAW.—With regard to the morbid conditions for which this operation is undertaken, it may be sufficient here to observe, that in no case can the operation be called justifiable in which the disease extends beyond the upper jaw-bone and the corresponding palate-bone, for unless the morbid growth be entirely removed, recurrence is inevitable, and no advantage is gained by the operation. It is undertaken for the removal of tumours of the antrum and of the alveolar margins, in all which cases the section for its removal must be made through healthy bone, and wide of the disease, so as to insure that the whole is removed. There are other cases in which the whole or part of the upper jaw has been removed for the purpose of giving access to disease behind, for example, to naso-pharyngeal polypi with extensive attachments.

In describing the operation for the excision of the entire upper jaw, we have to consider—(1.) what incisions through the soft parts will expose the tumour best, and with least deformity; (2.) what bony processes require to be divided, and where. Very various incisions have been recommended by various authors; some describing three, in various directions, forming flaps of different sizes, while others, again, are satisfied with a very small division of the upper lip into the nose, or even attempt removal of the bone without any incision through the skin at all. These discrepancies depend in great measure on different views of what constitutes excision of the upper jaw, the more complicated ones contemplating removal of the whole bone anatomically so called, including the floor of the orbit, while the less complicated ones are suitable for cases in which a much less extensive removal is required.

To remove the whole bone, an incision (Fig. xxvii. A) of the skin must extend from the angle of the mouth upwards and outwards in a slightly curved direction with its convexity downwards, as far on the malar bone as half an inch outside of the outer angle of the eye. The flaps must then be raised in both directions, the inner one specially dissected off the bones, so as to expose thoroughly the nasal cavity. It is of great importance thoroughly to display the floor of the orbit, so that the attachment of the orbital fascia may be accurately cut through, the inferior oblique muscle divided at its origin, and the eye and the fat of the orbit cautiously raised from its floor.

132

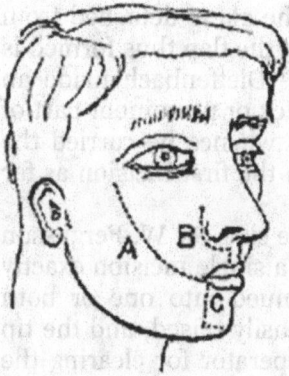

Fig. xxvii.[105]

Three processes of bone then require attention and division.

(1.) The articulation with the opposite bone in the hard palate. To divide this, one incisor tooth at least must be drawn, the soft palate divided by a knife to prevent laceration, and the thick alveolar portion sawn through in a longitudinal direction from before backwards.

(2.) The articulation with the malar bone at the upper angle of the incision through the skin. This must be notched with a small saw in a direction corresponding to the articulation, and then wrenched asunder by a pair of strong bone-pliers.

(3.) The nasal process of the upper jaw must now be divided by the pliers, one limb of which is cautiously inserted into the orbit, the other into the nose. If the disease extends high up in this process, it may be necessary partially to separate the corresponding nasal bone, and thus reach the suture between the nasal process and the frontal bone. The pliers must now be inserted into the groove already made by the saw on the hard palate, and the separation continued to the full extent backwards. A comparatively slight force exerted on the tumour either by the hand, or (when the tumour is small) by a pair of strong claw forceps, will suffice to break down the posterior attachments of the bone and remove it entire. The necessary laceration of the soft parts behind is so far an advantage, as it lessens the risk of hæmorrhage from the posterior palatine vessels.

The hæmorrhage from this operation was at one time much dreaded, but is rarely excessive; very few vessels require ligature, except those divided in the early stages in making the skin flaps; the hollow left should be stuffed with lint, which may be soaked in the perchloride of iron should there be any oozing.

The incisions recommended for this operation have been very various, and a knowledge of some of them may occasionally be useful, on account of specialities in the shape and size of the tumour. Liston "entered the bistoury over the external angular process of the frontal bone, and carried it down through the cheek to the corner of the mouth. Then the knife is to be pushed through the integument to the

---

[105] Diagram of operations on the jaws:—a, incision for removal of the whole upper jaw; b, incision for removal of alveolar portion and antrum; c, incision for removing the larger half of lower jaw; the opposite side is the one supposed to be operated on, and the incision is crossing the symphysis and turning up at a right angle.

133

nasal process of the maxilla, the cartilage of the ala is detached from the bone, and lip cut through in the mesial line; the flap thus formed is to be dissected up and the bones divided."[106] Dieffenbach made an incision through the upper lip and along the back or prominent part of the nose, up towards the inner canthus, from whence he carried the knife along the lower eyelid, at a right angle to the first incision as far as the malar bone.

In cases where the tumour is of moderate size, Sir W. Fergusson found[107] it sufficient to divide the upper lip by a single incision exactly in the middle line, this incision to be continued into one or both nostrils, if required. The ala of the nose is so easily raised, and the tip so moveable as to give great facilities to the operator for clearing the bone even to the floor of the orbit.

In cases where the tumour is larger, or the bones more extensively affected, Sir W. Fergusson preferred an extension of the foregoing incision (Fig. xxvii. B) upwards along the edge of the nose almost to the angle of the eye, and thence at a right angle along the lower eyelid, as far as may be necessary, even to the zygoma. The advantages claimed for such procedures are that the deformity is less and the vessels are divided at their terminal extremities.

2. EXCISION OF THE LOWER JAW.—Removal of portions, greater or smaller, of the lower jaw, for tumours, simple or malignant, are now operations of very frequent occurrence, while in some few cases the whole bone has been removed at both its articulations.

The operative procedures vary much, according to the amount of bone requiring removal, and also the position of the portion to be excised.

(1.) *Of a portion only of one side of the body of the bone.*—This is perhaps the simplest form of operation, and is frequently required for tumours, specially for epulis.

Incision.—If the parts are tolerably lax and the tumour small, a single incision just at the lower edge of the bone, of a length rather greater than the piece of bone to be removed, will suffice; this will divide the facial artery, which must be tied or compressed,[108] while the surgeon, dissecting on the tumour, separates the flaps in front, cutting upwards into the mouth, and then detaches the mylohyoid below, and clears the bone freely from mucous membrane. He then, with a narrow saw, notches the bone beyond the tumour at each side, and, introducing strong bone-pliers into the notches, is enabled to separate

---

[106] Operative Surgery, p. 265.

[107] Lancet, July 1, 1865.

[108] Temporary compression of the facial can be easily managed, in cases where it is of much importance to avoid loss of blood, by passing a needle from the outside through the skin above the vessel, then under the vessel, and out again through the skin below. A figure-of-eight suture can then be thrown round both ends of the needle, and the artery thus thoroughly compressed.

the required portion. The wound is then stitched up, and a very rapid cure generally results with very little deformity, as the cicatrix is in shadow. If from the size of the tumour more room is needed, it can easily be got by an additional incision from the angle of the mouth joining the former.

To prevent deformity, which is apt to result from the centre of the chin crossing the middle line, it is often a wise precaution to have a silver plate prepared fitting the molar teeth of both jaws on the sound side, and thus acting as a splint. Such a precaution may be required in any operation in which the lower jaw is sawn through.

N.B.—There are certain cases in which the epulis is small and confined to the alveolar margin, in which an attempt may be made to retain the base of the jaw entire, and remove the tumour without any incision of the skin. The mucous membrane on both sides being carefully dissected from the affected part, the bone may be sawn as before, but only through the alveolar portion, the groves of the saw converging as they penetrate, then by a pair of strong curved bone-pliers, the affected alveolar portion is to be scooped out without injuring the base. This proceeding, which has been practised by Syme, Fergusson, Pollock, the author in many cases, and others, leaves no deformity, but, it must be owned, is much more liable to the risk of recurrence of the disease, and for this reason is strongly condemned by Gross.

Note.—In this, as in all other operations on the jaws, the very first thing to be done is to draw the teeth at the spots at which the saw is to be applied.

(2.) *Excision of a portion involving the Symphysis.*—Free access is of importance. The best incision is probably one which (Fig. xxvii. C) commences at the angle of the mouth opposite the healthy portion of jaw, extends down to the place at which the saw is to be applied and then along the base of the jaw past the middle line to the other point of section. The flap is to be thrown up and the bone cleared. The next point to be noticed is, that when, in clearing the bone behind, the muscles attached to the symphysis are divided, the tongue loses its support, and unless watched may tend to fall backwards, embarrassing respiration and even perhaps choking the patient. The tongue, being confided to a special assistant, must be drawn well forwards. Various plans have been devised for keeping it in position, as stitching it to the point of the patient's nose; putting a ligature into its apex, and fastening it to the cheek by a piece of strapping, and transfixing its roots with a harelip needle, used to stitch up a central incision in the chin. The tendency to retraction very soon ceases, new attachments are formed by the muscles, and after the first five or six days there is very little risk of the tongue giving rise to any untoward consequences by its displacement.

(3.) *Disarticulation of one, or both Joints.*—When the portion of bone implicated involves disarticulation for its complete removal, the difficulty of the operation is much increased. The remarkably strong attachments of the joint, especially the relation of the temporal muscle to the coronoid process, and the close proximity of large arteries and nerves, especially the internal maxillary artery and the lingual nerve, render this disarticulation very difficult.

The chief points to be attended to seem to be (1.) that the incision through the skin should extend quite up to the level of the articulation; (2.) that the bone should be sawn through at the other side of the tumour, and freely cleared from all its attachments, before any attempt be made at disarticulation, for by means of the tumour great leverage can be attained, so as to put the muscles on the stretch, and allow them to be safely divided; (3.) that the articulation should always be entered from the front, not from behind, and the inner side of the condyle should be very carefully cleaned, the surgeon cutting on the bone so as to avoid, if possible, the internal maxillary artery; (4.) free and early division of the attachment of the temporal muscle to the coronoid process.

Disarticulation of the entire bone has been very rarely performed.[109] If necessary, it can be performed without any incision into the mouth, by one semilunar sweep from one articulation to the other, passing along the lower margin of each side of the body, and just below the symphysis of the chin.

Disarticulation of the Ramus without opening into the cavity of the Mouth.—That this operation is possible, though it may not be often required, is shown by the following case by Mr. Syme. It was a tumour of the ramus, extending only as far forwards as the wisdom-tooth:—

"An incision was made from the zygomatic arch down along the posterior margin of the ramus, slightly curved with its convexity towards the ear, to a little way beyond the base of the jaw. The parotid gland and masseter muscle being dissected off the jaw, it was divided by cutting-pliers immediately behind the wisdom-tooth, after being notched with a saw. The ramus was then seized by a strong pair of tooth-forceps, and notwithstanding strong posterior attachments, was drawn outwards, its muscular connections divided and turned out entire. There was thus no wound of the mucous membrane of the mouth, the masseter and pterygoid muscles were not completely divided, and the facial artery was intact."[110]

Fergusson[111] holds that even the very largest tumours of the lower jaw may be successfully removed without opening into the orifice of the mouth at all by division of the lips. A large lunated incision below

---

[109] Syme, Contributions to the Path. and Practice of Surgery, p. 21; Carnochan of New York, Cases in Surgery.

[110] Contributions to the Path. and Prac. of Surgery, pp. 23, 24.

[111] Lancet, July 1, 1865.

136

the lower margin of the bone, with its ends extending upwards to within half an inch of the lips, will give free access, and yet avoid both hæmorrhage and deformity, as the labial artery and vein are not cut, and there is no trouble in readjusting the lips. Some tumours of lower jaw can be removed without any wound of skin.

CHAPTER VIII

OPERATIONS ON MOUTH AND THROAT

SALIVARY FISTULA, *Operation for.*—After a wound or abscess of the cheek, in which the parotid duct is implicated, a salivary fistula is very apt to remain. The saliva thus discharges in the cheek, giving rise to considerable annoyance, as well as injury to the digestion. It is by no means easy to cure this. Perhaps the best operation is the one of which a rude diagram is given (Fig. xxviii.). The duct (c) communicates with the fistula (d). One end of a thread, either silken or metallic, should be passed through the fistula, and then as far backwards as convenient through the cheek into the mouth; the needle should then be withdrawn, the thread being left in. The other end being threaded should then be re-inserted at the fistula, and carried forwards in a similar manner; the needle should be again unthreaded in the mouth and withdrawn; the two ends should then be tied pretty tightly inside, and allowed to make their way by ulceration into the cavity of the mouth. A passage will thus be obtained for the saliva into the mouth, and every possible precaution should be taken to enable the external wound to close.

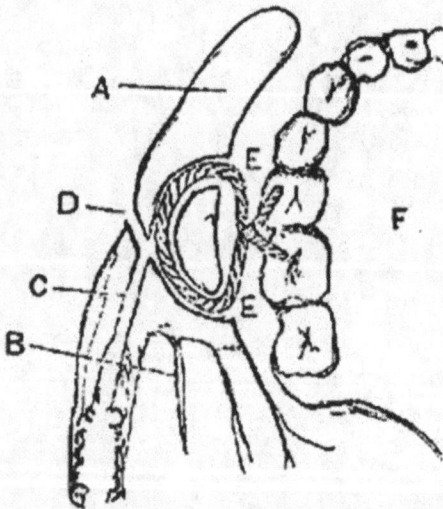

Fig. xxviii.[112]

EXCISION OF THE TONGUE, for malignant disease of the organ, may be either complete or partial. Complete excision affords a hope of permanent and complete relief from the disease, but it is an operation of extreme difficulty and danger. It may be performed in either of the following methods. The first is the only one in which absolute completeness of removal is insured.

---

[112] Rough diagram of operation for salivary fistula:—a, section of cheek close to buccal orifice; b, section of zygoma, muscles, etc.; c, the duct of the parotid; d, the fistulous opening of the cheek; E E, the thread knotted inside the mouth; f, the palate.

1. Syme's method of excision.—The patient being seated on a chair, chloroform was not administered, so that the blood might escape forwards, and not pass into the pharynx. The operation is thus described:[113]—

"Having extracted one of the front incisors, I cut through the middle of the lip and continued the incision down to the os hyoides, then sawed through the jaw in the same line, and insinuating my finger under the tongue as a guide to the knife, divided the mucous lining of the mouth, together with the attachment of the genio-hyoglossi. While the two halves of the bone were held apart, I dissected backwards, and cut through the hyoglossi, along with the mucous membrane covering them, so as to allow the tongue to be pulled forward, and bring into view the situation of the lingual arteries, which were cut and tied, first on one side, and then on the other. The process might now have been at once completed, had I not feared that the epiglottis might be implicated in the disease, which extended beyond the reach of my finger, and thus suffer injury from the knife if used without a guide. I therefore cut away about two-thirds of the tongue, and then being able to reach the os hyoides with my finger, retained it there while the remaining attachments were divided by the knife in my other hand close to the bone. Some small arterial branches having been tied, the edges of the wound were brought together and retained by silver sutures, except at the lowest part, where the ligatures were allowed to maintain a drain for the discharge of fluids from the cavity." The patient was able to swallow from a drinking-cup with a spout on the day following the operation, and was able to travel upwards of 200 miles within four weeks of the operation.

2. By the Écraseur.—Nunneley of Leeds has recorded cases in which he made a small incision through the skin, and mylohyoid and geniohyoid muscles, and through this passed a curved needle bearing the chain of the écraseur completely round the base of the tongue. In one case the chain was unsatisfactory, but strong whipcord was introduced as it was withdrawn, and tied with all possible force. The organ eventually sloughed away, with a cure which lasted at least for some months.

Sir James Paget operates as follows:—

The patient is placed under the influence of chloroform, and the mouth held widely open. The tongue is then drawn forwards, the mucous membrane and soft parts of the floor of the mouth, including the attachment of the genio-hyoglossi to the symphysis being divided close to the bone. The steel wire of an écraseur is then passed round its root as low down as possible, slowly tightened, and the tongue thus divided through its whole thickness in a very few minutes. The bleeding

---

[113] Lancet, Feb. 4, 1865.

is slight, being almost entirely from the parts cut with the knife. Recovery has been rapid in the recorded cases.[114]

To Dr. George Buchanan of Glasgow the credit is due of the invention of the operation of removal of the half of the tongue in the median line. In at least one instance the cure after five years is still permanent.

Partial excisions of the tongue are as unsatisfactory in their results as they are unsound in principle, yet many cases present themselves, in which, while the patient urges some operative measure for his relief, the tumour is so limited as not to warrant the exceedingly dangerous operation of complete excision.

Portions may be removed in various ways:—

1. By the knife. If in the apex, by a V-shaped incision; if in the lateral regions, by a bold free incision with a probe-pointed bistoury round the tumour.

2. By ligature, drawn as tightly as possible, and, if the portion included be large, in successive portions.

3. By the écraseur.

Mr. Furneaux Jordan has removed the whole tongue with success by means of two écraseurs worked at the same time.[115]

4. By the galvano-caustic wire.

5. The author has in nine cases removed the affected half of the tongue by means of the thermo-cautery, first splitting it in the middle line and then cutting through the base with a curved platinum knife at a low red heat. In one only was there any trouble from hæmorrhage, and all made good recoveries.

Mr. Barwell has recorded (Lancet, 1879, vol. i.) an easy, safe, and comparatively painless mode of removing the tongue by écraseurs.

Mr. Walter Whitehead,[116] of Manchester, has had a very large experience of an operation devised by himself, in which, after pulling the tongue well forward by a string previously introduced near its apex, and the mouth being held open by a gag, he detaches the organ from jaw and fauces by successive short snips with scissors, and then in same manner divides the muscles, tying or twisting the vessels as they bleed. His success has been very great by this method, though others who have tried it have sometimes found bleeding troublesome.

It is comparatively seldom now necessary to split the jaw and perform Syme's operation, and in all operations on the tongue the thermocautory (Paquelin's) is of great use.

Regnoli's method[117] may deserve a brief notice. A semilunar incision along the base of the jaw, from one angle to the other, detaches

---

[114] Med. Times and Gazette for Feb. 10, 1866.
[115] Lancet, April 20, 1872.
[116] Transactions International Medical Congress, 1881, vol. ii. p. 460.
[117] Gross's Surgery, vol. ii. p. 472.

the muscles and soft structures, and is thrown down; the tongue is then drawn through the opening, and can be freely dealt with either by knife or ligature. After removal the flap is replaced.

FISSURES IN THE PALATE.—The operations requisite for the cure of fissures in the soft and hard palates are so complicated in their details, that a small treatise would be required thoroughly to describe the various procedures.

Different cases vary so much in the nature and amount of their deformity, that at least five different sets of cases have been described. It is sufficient here merely to describe the absolutely essential principles of the operations for the cure of fissures of the hard and soft palate respectively.

In all operations on the palate, two conditions used to be considered requisite for success:—1. That the patient should have arrived at years of discretion, at twelve or fourteen years at least; that he be possessed of considerable firmness, and be extremely anxious for a cure, so as to give full and intelligent co-operation. 2. That for some days or weeks prior to the operation the mouth and palate should have been trained to open widely and to bear manipulation, without reflex action being excited. Professor Billroth of Vienna,[118] and Mr. Thomas Smith[119] of London, have had cases which prove the possibility of performing this operation in childhood, under chloroform, with the assistance, in the English cases, of a suitable gag, invented by Mr. Smith. The effect of the operation on the voice of the child has been very encouraging, as much more improvement takes place than in cases where the operation is performed late in life.

Fissure in the soft palate only appears as a triangular cleft, the apex of which is above, the base being a line between the points of the bifid uvula, which are widely separated. To cure this it is required—

1. That the edges of the fissure should be brought together without strain or tightness. In small fissures this can generally be done easily enough; but where the fissure is extensive, some means must be used to relieve tension. For this, Sir William Fergusson long ago proposed the division of the palatal muscles, the levator, tensor, and palato-pharyngeus muscle of each side. The incisions in the palate for this purpose certainly aid apposition, but many surgeons entertain doubts whether the division of the muscles has much to do with the good result, and believe that the simple incisions in the mucous membrane, in a proper direction, are all that is required (see Fig. xxix.).

---

[118] Langenbeck, Archiv, ii. p. 657.
[119] Med. Chir. Trans. for 1867-8.

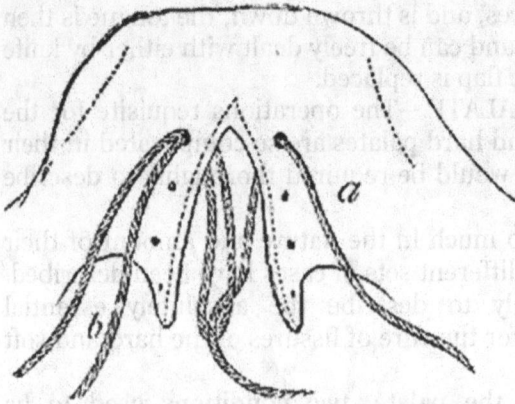

Fig. xxix.[120]

2. That the edges of the fissure be made raw, so as to afford surfaces which will readily unite. Complicated instruments, such as knives of various strange shapes, have been devised for this purpose; an ordinary cataract knife, very sharp, and set on a long handle is perhaps the best. It greatly facilitates the section if the parts are tense, so the point of the uvula should be seized by an ordinary pair of spring forceps, and drawn across the roof of the mouth, while the knife should enter in the middle line, a little above the apex of the fissure, and make the cut downwards as in harelip.

3. That sutures should be inserted to keep the edges in apposition, yet not so tightly as to cause ulceration. They may be either of metal, silver being preferable, or of fine silk well waxed. The metallic sutures are now generally preferred. Some dexterity is required in their introduction, and various instruments have been devised; the best seems to be a needle with a short curve fixed on a long handle, which should be entered on the (patient's) left side of the fissure in front, and brought out on the right side.

If silk sutures be used, the chief difficulty, that of passing the thread through the second side from behind forwards, can be avoided in the following manner.[121] A curved needle is passed through one side of the fissure, and then towards the middle line, till its point is seen through the cleft. One of the ends of the thread is then seized by a long pair of forceps, and drawn through the cleft; the needle is then withdrawn, leaving the thread through the palate, and both ends are brought outside at the angle of the mouth. Another needle is then passed through a corresponding point at the opposite side of the palate, till its point again appears at the cleft; this time a double loop of the thread is also brought out through the cleft by the forceps into the mouth. If then the single thread of the first ligature which is in the cleft be passed through the loop of the second one also in the cleft, it is easy, by withdrawing the loop through the palate, to finish the stitch (see Fig.

---

[120] Diagram of staphyloraphy, chiefly to illustrate the passing of the threads:—a, the first thread; b, the second. The dotted line at edge of fissure shows amount to be removed; the other dotted lines showing size and position of the incision through the mucous membrane above.

[121] Holmes's Surgery, vol. ii. pp. 504-513.

xxix.). All the stitches should be passed and their position approved before any one be tied, and it is most convenient to secure them from above downwards. To prevent confusion, each pair of threads after being inserted should be left very long, and brought up to a coronet fixed on the brow, which is fitted with several pairs of hooks numbered for easy reference. This will prevent twisting of the threads or any mistake in tying.

FISSURE OF THE HARD PALATE.—This may vary in extent from a very slight cleft in the middle line behind, up to a complete separation of the two halves of the jaw, including even the alveolar process in front, and sometimes complicated with harelip.

To close such fissures by operation is difficult, as the breadth of the cleft is so great as to prevent the apposition of the edges when prepared, without such extreme tension as quite prevents any hope of union. Through the researches of Avery, Warren, Langenbeck, and others, a method has been discovered of closing such fissures by operation, which, though certainly not easy, is, when properly performed, generally successful.

Operation.—In addition to the usual paring of the edges of the cleft, an incision is made on each side of the palate, extending "from the canine tooth in front to the last molar behind,"[122] along the alveolar ridge (Fig. xxx.). The whole flap between the cleft and this incision on each side is then to be raised from the bone by a blunt rounded instrument slightly curved. With this the whole mucous membrane and as much of the periosteum as possible should be completely raised from the bone, attachments for nourishment of the flap being left in front and behind where the vessels enter.

Fig. xxx.[123]

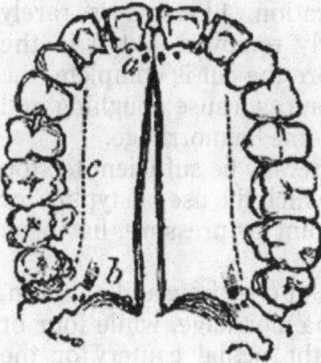

The flaps thus raised will be found to come together in the middle line, sometimes even to overlap, and, when united by suture, form a new palate at a lower level than the fissure, experience having shown that in cases of fissure the arch of the palate is always much higher than usual. The flaps do not slough, being well supplied with blood, unless they have been injured in their separation.

[122] Edinburgh Medical Journal for Jan. 1865, Mr. Annandale's instructive paper on "Cleft Palate."

[123] Diagram of fissure of hard palate:—a, anterior palatine foramina; b, posterior palatine foramina with groove for artery; c, incisions requisite to free the soft structures.

The edges must be carefully united by various points of metallic suture, and the fissure of the soft palate closed at the same sitting, unless the patient has lost much blood, or is very much exhausted with the pain. The stitches may be left in for a week, or even ten days, unless they are exciting much irritation. The patient must exercise great self-control and caution in the character of his food and his manner of eating for ten days or a fortnight after the operation.

EXCISION OF TONSILS.—To remove the whole tonsil is of course impossible in the living body, the operation to which the name of excision is given being only the shaving off of a redundant and projecting portion. When properly performed it is a very safe, and in adults a very easy operation, but in children it is sometimes rendered exceedingly difficult by their struggles, combined with the movements of the tongue and the insufficient access through the small mouth. Many instruments have been devised for the purpose of at once transfixing and excising the projecting portion; some of them are very ingenious and complicated. By far the best and safest method of removing the redundant portion is to seize it with a volsellum, and then cut it off by a single stroke of a probe-pointed curved bistoury; cutting from above downwards, and being careful to cut parallel with the great vessels.

The ordinary volsellum is much improved for this purpose by the addition of a third hook in each tonsil placed between the others, with a shorter curve, and slightly shorter; this ensures the safe holding of the fragment removed, and prevents the risk of its falling down the throat of the patient.

If both tonsils are enlarged they should both be operated on at the same sitting, and the pain is so slight that even children frequently make little objection to the second operation. Bleeding is rarely troublesome if the portion be at once fairly removed, but if in the patient's struggles the hook should slip before the cut is complete, the partially detached portion will irritate the fauces, cause coughing and attempts to vomit, and sometimes a troublesome hæmorrhage.

The plentiful use of cold water will generally be sufficient to stop the bleeding, though cases are on record in which the use of styptics, or even the temporary closure of a bleeding point by pressure, has been necessary.

M. Guersant has operated on more than one thousand children, with only three cases of any trouble from hæmorrhage, while four or five out of fifteen adults required either the actual cautery or the sesqui-chloride of iron.[124]

---

[124] Holmes's Diseases of Children, p. 555.

CHAPTER IX

OPERATIONS ON AIR PASSAGES

OPERATIONS ON THE LARYNX AND TRACHEA.—The great air passage may be opened at three different situations, and to the operations at these different places the following names have been given:—

Laryngotomy, when the opening is made in the interval between the cricoid and thyroid cartilages, through the crico-thyroid membrane.

Laryngo-tracheotomy, when the cricoid cartilage and the upper ring of the trachea are divided.

Tracheotomy, when the trachea itself is opened by the division of two, three, or more rings.

Of these the last, tracheotomy, is by far the most frequent, important, difficult, and dangerous, and requires a very detailed description. Chassaignac[125] says "the only really rational operation for the opening of the air passages by the surgeon is tracheotomy."

TRACHEOTOMY.—*Anatomy.*—Between the cricoid cartilage and the level of the upper border of the sternum, the middle line of the neck is occupied by the upper portion of the trachea. Its depth from the surface varies, gradually increasing as the trachea descends, and varying very much according to the fatness, muscularity, and length of the neck. It is, however, almost subcutaneous at the commencement below the cricoid, and on the level of the sternum it is in most cases at least an inch from the surface, in many much deeper. Again, its length varies, even in the adult, from two and a half to three, or even four inches. This is important, as affecting the simplicity of the operation, which, as a rule, is easier the longer the neck is.

The trachea has most important and complicated anatomical relations—some constant, others irregular.

1. The carotid arteries and jugular veins lie at either side, but, where these are regular in their distribution, do not practically interfere in a well-conducted operation.

2. The thyroid gland lies in close relation to the trachea, one lobe being at each side (Fig. xxxi. B B), and the isthmus of the thyroid crosses the trachea just over the second and third cartilaginous rings. In fat vascular necks, or where the thyroid is enlarged it may occupy a much larger portion of the trachea. The position of the isthmus practically divides the trachea into two portions in which it is possible to perform tracheotomy. Both have their advocates, but the balance of

---

[125] Leçons sur la Trachéotomie, p. 10.

145

authority tends to support the operation below the thyroid. A separate notice of each will be required immediately.

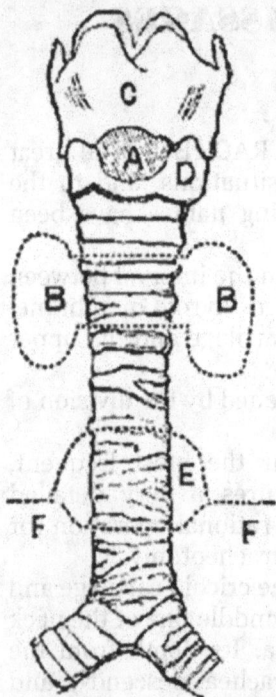

Fig. xxxi.[126]

3. The muscles in relation to the trachea are the sterno-hyoid and sterno-thyroid of each side. The latter are the broadest, are in close contact across the trachea by the inner edges below, but gradually diverge as they ascend the neck. In thick-set, muscular necks, however, they are in close contact for a considerable distance, and require to be separated to give access to the trachea.

The arteries are in most cases unimportant; no named branch of any size ought to be divided in the operation. However, occasionally very free bleeding may result from the division of an abnormal thyroidea ima running up the trachea to the thyroid body from the innominate, or even from the aorta itself.

The veins are very numerous and irregularly distributed. There is generally a large transverse communicating branch between the superior thyroid veins just above the isthmus. The isthmus itself has a large venous plexus over it. Below the isthmus the veins converge into one trunk (or sometimes two parallel ones) lying right in front of the trachea.

4. The last anatomical point which may give trouble in normal necks is the thymus, which is present in children below the age of two, and covers the lower end of the trachea just above the level of the sternum. Where this is not only not diminished, but enlarged, as it sometimes is in unhealthy children, it may give a very great deal of trouble, rolling out at the wound and greatly embarrassing proceedings.

Abnormalities are very various and sometimes very dangerous: vessels crossing the trachea, as the innominate did in Macilwain's case,[127] or where two brachiocephalic trunks are present, as recorded by Chassaignac.[128] One of the most frequent dangers to be guarded

---

[126] Rough diagram of larynx and trachea:—A, crico-thyroid space, laryngotomy; B B, dotted outline of thyroid isthmus and lobes, defines the upper and lower positions for tracheotomy; C, thyroid—D, cricoid cartilages; E, dotted outline of thymus gland in child of two years; F F, outline of clavicles and jugular fossa.

[127] Surgical Observations, p. 335. See also Harrison On the Arteries, vol. i. p. 16.

[128] Leçons sur la Trachéotomie, p. 9.

against is a possible dilatation of the aorta or aneurism of the arch. This may very possibly, as happened in one case to the author, give rise to suffocative paroxysms from its pressure on the recurrent laryngeal nerves. Tracheotomy may be deemed necessary, and there is a great risk, unless proper precautions be taken, of wounding the aorta, where it passes upwards in the jugular fossa. In the author's case the vessel had actually to be pushed downwards by the pulp of the forefinger while the trachea was opened, the knife being guided on the back of the nail of the same finger.

THE OPERATION.—In a work of this kind it would be utterly impossible to go at all into the subject of what diseases, injuries, etc., warrant or require the operation. It is enough to describe the various methods of operating, their dangers and difficulties.

1. *The operation above the isthmus of the thyroid.*—A spot about a quarter or half of an inch in vertical diameter between the cricoid cartilage (Fig. xxxi.) and thyroid isthmus.

Advantages.—It is near the surface, the vessels are few and comparatively small. It is most suitable in cases of aneurism.

Professor Spence[129] gives his sanction to the high operation in adults with thick short necks when the operation is performed for ulceration or papilloma of larynx or for spasm from aneurism, the low operation being still best in cases of croup or diphtheria.

Disadvantages.—The space is too small, requires very considerable disturbance of the thyroid isthmus, or actual division of it. It is too near the point where the disease is; so much so, that in most cases of croup or diphtheria it would be perfectly useless. However, if required, or if the operation lower down be contra-indicated, this may be performed easily enough. A straight incision being made in the middle line about one inch and a half in length, expose the upper ring by careful dissection, if possible draw aside the veins, and depress the thyroid isthmus, divide the rings thus exposed, and introduce the tube.

The operation below the isthmus.—This, though more difficult in its performance, is a much more scientific and satisfactory operation. Considerable coolness and a thorough knowledge of the anatomy of the part are absolutely required.

The patient being in the recumbent posture, the shoulders should be well raised, and the head held back so as to extend the windpipe, and thus bring it as near as possible to the surface. A pillow, or the arm of an assistant, behind the neck will be of service.

N.B.—Be careful lest too great extension by an anxious assistant, accompanied by closure of the mouth, should choke the patient (whose breathing is of course already much embarrassed) before the operation be begun.

Chloroform may occasionally be given, and, if well borne,

---

[129] Lectures on Surgery, 3d ed., vol. ii. p. 900.

renders the operation very much easier than it would otherwise be. An incision must then be made exactly in the median line of the neck, from a little below the cricoid cartilage, almost to the upper edge of the sternum; at first it should be through skin only, then the veins will be seen, probably turgid with dark blood; the larger ones should be drawn aside, if necessary divided, the bleeding stopped by gentle pressure. The deep fascia must then be cautiously divided, great care being taken to keep exactly in the middle line, and the contiguous edges of sterno-thyroid muscles separated from each other by the handle of the knife. A quantity of loose connective tissue, containing numerous small veins, must now be pushed aside, the thyroid isthmus pressed upwards, still with the handle of the knife. The forefinger must then be used to distinguish the rings of the trachea. If there is much convulsive movement of the larynx and trachea, they should be fixed by the insertion of a small sharp hook with a short curve, just below the cricoid cartilage, and this should be confided to an assistant. The surgeon should then, with the forefinger of his left hand, fix the trachea, and open it by a straight sharp-pointed scalpel, boldly thrusting it through the rings with a jerk or stab, the back of the knife being below, and divide two or three of the rings from below upwards. Any attempt to enter the trachea slowly with a blunt knife or trocar will probably be unsuccessful, as the rings, especially in children, give way before the knife, which merely approximates the sides of the trachea without opening it.

Question of Hæmorrhage.—It is often a question of some importance, and one which sometimes it is not easy to settle, how far attempts should be made completely to arrest the venous hæmorrhage before opening the trachea.

On the one hand, if not arrested, besides the risk of weakening the patient, we have to dread the much more serious complication of the admission of blood into the wound. And this is very serious in a patient whose respiration has already been much impeded, whose lungs are probably engorged, and who has certainly, by the mere existence of a wound in his trachea, lost the power of coughing properly; it must never be forgotten that a quantity of blood so trifling as to be at once ejected by a single cough in the case of a healthy chest, may be a fatal obstacle to respiration in one already weakened by disease. Thus any well-marked arterial hæmorrhage from cut branches, or from the isthmus of the thyroid, must certainly be arrested prior to opening the trachea. Besides this, blood once having entered the bronchi is apt to extend into their smaller ramifications and prove a cause of death, by acting as a local irritation, and setting up intra-lobular suppurative pneumonia. The author has found this to be the case both after tracheotomy and still more frequently in suicide by cut throat.

But, on the other hand, it is equally true that there is almost always a considerable amount of oozing from small venous radicles divided during the operation, which depends simply on the great venous engorgement resulting from the obstruction to the respiration, so that while to attempt to tie every point would be simply endless, we may be almost certain that the oozing will cease whenever the trachea is opened, and respiration fairly improved. Slight pressure on the wound is generally sufficient to stop the bleeding till the venous engorgement has disappeared.

Of late years many tracheotomies have been done bloodlessly by use of the thermo-cautery, for division of the soft parts, but the subsequent sloughing of the wound is a great objection to this method.

In cases of extreme urgency, all such minor considerations as suppression of venous oozing must be ignored, and the trachea simply opened as rapidly as possible. I had once to perform the operation after respiration had entirely ceased, and no pulse could be felt at the wrist, with no assistance except that of a female attendant. Merely feeling that no large arterial branch was in the way, I cut straight through all the tissues, opened the trachea, and commenced artificial respiration. The patient eventually recovered.

Question of Tubes, etc.—Once the trachea is opened, the next question is, How is the opening to be kept pervious? For the moment the handle of the scalpel is to be inserted in the wound, so as to stretch it transversely; this will probably suffice to allow of the escape of any foreign body. But where, to admit air, the wound is to be kept open, how is this to be done? It used to be advised that an elliptical portion of the wall of the trachea be removed; this, though succeeding well enough for a time, was unscientific, as the wound always tended to cicatrise, and ended of course in permanent narrowing of the canal of the trachea. It may be necessary thus to excise a portion of the trachea, in cases where it is very intolerant of the presence of a tube. Such a case is recorded by Sir J. Fayrer of Calcutta.[130] Not much better is the proposal to insert a silk ligature in each side of the wound, and by pulling these apart thus mechanically to open the wound. This also is evidently a merely temporary expedient.

Various canulæ and tubes have been proposed. The ones recommended by the older surgeons had all one great fault; they were much too small, and were many of them straight, and thus liable to displacement. The smallness of their bore was their greatest objection, and Mr. Liston conferred a great benefit on surgery by his insisting upon the introduction of tubes with a larger bore, and with a proper curve, so as thoroughly to enter the trachea. The tube ought to be large enough to admit all the air required by the lungs, without hurrying the respiration in the least.

There is a mistake made in the construction of many of the tubes

---

[130] Clinical Surgery in India (1866), p. 143.

even of the present day; the outer opening is large and full, while for convenience of insertion the tube tapers down to an inner opening, admitting perhaps not one-half as much air as the outer one does.

It must be remembered that for some days there is great risk of the tube becoming occluded, by frothy blood or mucus, especially in cases of croup, and in children. To prevent this a double canula will be found of great service, providing only that it be remembered that the inner canula, not the outer merely, is to be made large enough to breathe through, and that the inner should project slightly beyond the outer one.

The inner one can thus be removed at intervals and cleansed, by the nurse, without any risk of exciting spasm or dyspnœa by its absence and reintroduction.

After-treatment.—The after-treatment of a case in which tracheotomy has been performed demands great care and many precautions. For the first day or two the constant presence of an experienced nurse or student is always necessary to insure the patency of the tube. The temperature of the room should be equable and high, and it seems of importance that the air should be kept moist as well as warm by the use of abundance of steam.

A piece of thin gauze, or other light protective material, should be placed over the mouth of the tube, to prevent the entrance of foreign bodies.

In cases where the operation has been performed for some temporary inflammatory closure of the air passage, retention of the tube for a few days may suffice. It may then be removed, but it must be remembered that the wound will generally close with great rapidity, so that it is as well to be quite sure of the patency of the natural passage before the artificial one is allowed to close by the removal of the tube.

In cases where from long-standing disease or severe accident the larynx is rendered totally unfit for work, and the tube has to be worn during the rest of the patient's life, care must be taken (1.) lest the tube do not fit accurately, in which case it may ulcerate in various directions, even into the great vessels;[131] (2.) lest the tube become worn, and lest the part within the windpipe fall into the trachea and suffocate the patient.[132]

LARYNGOTOMY.—As a temporary expedient in cases of great urgency, where proper instruments and assistants are not at hand, laryngotomy is occasionally useful, though from the want of space without encroaching on the cartilages of the larynx, and from its close proximity to the disease, laryngotomy is by no means a suitable or permanently successful operation.

---

[131] Mr. John Wood, Path. Soc. Trans., vol. xi. p. 20.
[132] South's Chelius, vol. ii. p. 400; and case recorded by Spence, in Ed. Med. Journal, for August 1862.

In the adult, especially in males with long spare necks, the operation itself is exceedingly easy to perform. The crico-thyroid space (Fig. xxxi. a) is so distinctly shown by the prominence of the thyroid cartilage, and is so superficial that it is quite easy to open it in the middle line with a common penknife, there being merely the skin and the crico-thyroid membrane to be cut through, with very rarely any vessel of any size. The opening can then be kept patent by a quill or a small piece of flat wood. This simple operation has in many cases, where a foreign body has filled up the box of the larynx, succeeded in saving life, and even in cases of disease I have known it useful in giving time for the subsequent performance of tracheotomy.

Easy as it appears and really is, cases are on record in which the thyro-hyoid space has been opened instead of the crico-thyroid, such operations being of course perfectly useless.

The incision is best made transversely.

LARYNGO-TRACHEOTOMY.—This modification consists in opening the air passage by the division of the cricoid cartilage vertically in the middle line, along with one or two of the upper rings of the trachea.

It seems to combine all the dangers with none of the advantages of the other methods of operating. It is close to the disease, involves cutting a cartilage of the larynx, and almost certain wounding of the isthmus of the thyroid; and it is not easy to see what corresponding advantages it has over tracheotomy in the usual position.

THYROTOMY is an operation by which the larynx is opened in the middle line by a vertical incision, and its halves separated, while any morbid growths are excised from the cords or ventricles. The merits and dangers of this operation have been discussed at length by Mr. Durham[133] and Dr. Morell Mackenzie.[134]

LARYNGECTOMY OR EXCISION OF THE LARYNX, first performed by Dr. Heron Watson in 1866, has been lately frequently performed for carcinoma and sarcoma. Each case presents its own difficulties, which vary according to the amount and extent of the disease for which it is done.

The trachea must be divided and tamponed by a Trendelenburg canula, after which the larynx must be carefully dissected out. The immediate mortality, i.e. in first ten days, is fifty per cent., and Dr. Gross holds that life has not been prolonged by the operation.[135]

ŒSOPHAGOTOMY.—This operation is very rarely required, and has as yet been performed only for the removal of foreign bodies impacted in the œsophagus, and interfering with respiration and deglutition. To cut upon the flaccid empty œsophagus in the living body

---

[133] Med. Chir. Transactions of London, 1872.
[134] British Med. Journal (Nos. 643, 644), 1873.
[135] Gross's Surgery, 6th ed., vol. ii. p. 342.

would be an extremely difficult and dangerous operation, from the manner in which it lies concealed behind the larynx, and in close contact with the great vessels. When it is distended by a foreign body, and specially if the foreign body has well-marked angles, the operation is not nearly so difficult. It has now been performed in forty-three cases at least, of which eight or nine have proved fatal. Seven, along with another in which he himself performed it with success, were recorded by Mr. Cock of Guy's Hospital.[136] Three others were performed by Mr. Syme, with a successful result. Of the seven cases collected by Mr. Cock only two died, one of pneumonia, the other of gangrene of the pharynx.

Operation.—Unless there is a very decided projection of the foreign body on the right, the left side of the neck should be chosen, as the œsophagus normally lies rather on the left of the middle line. An incision similar to that required for ligature of the carotid above the omohyoid should be made over the inner edge of the sterno-mastoid muscle; with it as a guide, the omohyoid may be sought and drawn downwards and inwards, the sheath of the vessels exposed and drawn outwards, the larynx slightly pushed across to the right, the thyroid gland drawn out of the way by a blunt hook, the superior thyroid either avoided or tied. The œsophagus is then exposed, and if the foreign body is large, it is easily recognised; if the foreign body be small, a large probang with a globular ivory head should then be passed from the fauces down to the obstruction; this will distend the walls of the œsophagus, and make it a much more easy and safe business to divide them to the required extent. The wound in the œsophagus should be longitudinal, and at first not larger than is required to admit the finger, on which as a guide the forceps may be introduced to remove the foreign body, or, if necessary, a probe-pointed bistoury still further to dilate the wound.

For some days or even weeks the patient must be fed through an elastic catheter introduced through the nose and retained, or by an ordinary stomach-tube through the mouth. In introducing the latter there is always a risk of opening the wound. No special sutures for the wound in the œsophagus are required, nor is it advisable too closely to sew up the external wound.

---

[136] Guy's Hospital Reports for 1858.

CHAPTER X

OPERATIONS ON THORAX

EXCISION OF MAMMA.—When the whole breast is to be removed, two incisions, inclosing an elliptical portion of skin along with the nipple, must be made in the direction of the fibres of the pectoralis muscle. The distance between the incisions at their broadest must depend upon the nature of the disease for which the operation is performed, and the extent to which the skin is involved; in every case the whole nipple should be removed. The incisions should, if possible, be parallel with the fibres of the pectoralis major, and extend across the full diameter of the breast. During the operation the arm should be extended so as to stretch both skin and muscle. The lower flap should be first raised and dissected downwards, with care that the cuts are made in the subcutaneous fat, and wide of the disease; the upper flap is then thrown open, and the edge of the gland raised, so that the fibres of the pectoralis are exposed below it. These should be cleanly dissected, so as to insure removal of the whole gland.

Any bleeding during the operation can easily be checked by the fingers of an assistant, and if the arteries entering the gland from the axilla be divided last, they can be at once secured. If there are many bleeding points, the application of cold for a few hours before the wound is finally closed is a wise precaution.

The requisite stitches may be inserted while the patient is under chloroform, but not tightened. The arm should then be brought down to the side, and a folded towel laid over the wound after it is finally closed. Great benefit results from the free use of drainage-tubes in most cases; for this purpose a dependent opening in the lower flap is often made.

Surgeons now operate even when the axillary glands are diseased, and by a very free dissection and removal, even in hopeless-looking cases, life may be prolonged. To insure the removal of the lymphatic vessels as well as the glands, it is best not to separate the breast at its axillary margin, but keep it attached by the tail of lymphatics surrounded by fat, which will lead up to the glands. Section of the great pectoral muscle will aid the dissection.

When the tumour is very large, and the skin has been much stretched and undermined, more complicated incisions may be necessary; these must be governed a good deal by the presence and positions of adhesions or ulcerations of the skin. The best direction, when the surgeon has his choice, that these

153

incisions can take, is that of radii from the nipple, bisecting the flaps made by the original elliptical incision.

N.B.—In operating for malignant disease, the one paramount consideration is that all the disease be excised, however curious, inconvenient, or awkward, even insufficient, the flaps may look. Partial excisions are worse than useless.

Paracentesis Thoracis, for the relief of pleurisy, acute and chronic, and empyema, is an operation of extreme simplicity.

The proper selection of cases, the settling of the suitable position for the tapping, and the choosing of the suitable time for it, are more difficult, and not within the scope of the present work. On these subjects much information may be obtained from the papers of Dr. Bowditch of Boston, of Dr. Hughes and Mr. Cock,[137] and an exceedingly interesting and valuable paper by Dr. Warburton Begbie.[138]

Where is it to be performed? Not above the sixth rib, else the opening is not sufficiently dependent; very rarely below the eighth on the right side, and the ninth on the left. The intercostal space generally bulges outwards if fluid is present, and this bulging acts as an aid to diagnosis. As the intercostal artery lies under the lower edge of the upper rib in each space, the trocar should be entered not higher than the middle of the space; and because the artery is largest near the spine, and also the space is there deeply covered with muscle, the tapping should never be behind the angle of the rib. In most of the manuals we are told to select a spot midway between the sternum and spine for the puncture; but Bowditch, Cock, and Begbie, who have had large experience, prefer, and I believe rightly, a position considerably behind this, an inch or two below the angle of the scapula, between the seventh and eighth, or between the eighth and ninth ribs.

The operation may be performed with a simple trocar and canula, round, about an eighth of an inch in diameter, and at least two inches in length. The point must be sharp, and it must be pushed in with considerable quickness, so as to penetrate, not merely push forwards, the pleura, which may be tough, and thicker than usual. Once the skin is pierced, the instrument must be directed obliquely upwards, so as to make the opening and position of the trocar dependent. When the trocar is withdrawn the fluid may be allowed to flow so long as it keeps in a full equable stream; whenever it becomes jerky and spasmodic, the canula should be removed before the sucking noise of air entering the chest is heard.

In more chronic cases, where the quantity of fluid is large, and especially if it is thick and curdy, the exhausting syringe of Mr. Bowditch is an improvement on the simple trocar and canula.

It consists of a powerful syringe, which fits accurately to the

[137]Both in Guy's Hospital Reports, second series, vol. ii.
[138] Edinburgh Medical Journal for June 1866.

154

trocar with which the puncture is made. There is a stop-cock between the trocar and syringe, and another at right angles to the syringe. The trocar being introduced, it is held firmly in position by an assistant, by means of a strong cross handle; the first stop-cock is then opened, and the syringe worked slowly till it is filled with fluid through the trocar, the other delivery stop-cock being closed. The first is then closed, and the second opened; the syringe is then emptied through the second into a basin. By a repetition of this process, the fluid can be removed at pleasure, without any risk of the entrance of air.

Dieulafoy's aspirateur, which the author has now used in a very large number of cases, will be found the best method yet devised of safely removing the fluid in cases of serous effusion. But in severe cases of empyema the pus is sure to be reproduced in the great majority, and then a free incision, with strict antiseptic precautions, will be needed, and subsequent free drainage.

The author has used with great benefit silver tubes, like long narrow   trachea-tubes, with broad shields, to insure free drain.

155

CHAPTER XI

OPERATIONS ON ABDOMEN

PARACENTESIS ABDOMINIS.—To withdraw fluid from the abdominal cavity is an exceedingly simple operation in itself, though certain precautions are necessary to render it safe.

Trocar.—The usual instrument used to be a simple round canula with a trocar, the point of which should be very sharp, and in the shape of a three-sided pyramid. It should be about three inches in length, and a quarter of an inch in diameter. It may for convenience have an india-rubber tube fixed to its side or end, for the purpose of conveying the fluid to the pail or basin, but any other additions or alterations have not been improvements. Lately surgeons have been diminishing the size of the tube so as to withdraw the fluid more slowly, and taking many precautions to insure the wound being kept aseptic.

Where to tap.—In the linea alba, midway between the umbilicus and pubes, or rather nearer the umbilicus. Here, there are no muscles nor vessels, the opening is a dependent one, and the bladder is quite out of the way of injury.

N.B.—It is a wise precaution, in every case where there is a possibility of doubt as to the state of the bladder, to pass a catheter. I have myself known at least one case in which a surgeon was asked to tap an over-distended bladder, as a case of ascites.

The Operation.—As there is great risk of syncope coming on during the operation, from the sudden relief to the pressure on the organs, a broad flannel bandage should be applied to the belly, the ends of which are split into three at each side, and crossed and interlaced behind. An assistant should stand at each side to make gradual pressure by pulling on the ends of the bandage, thus assisting the flow, and maintaining the pressure. A hole should be cut in the bandage at the spot where the puncture is to be made, and the trocar inserted by one firm push, without any preliminary incision, unless the patient is inordinately fat. As the trocar is withdrawn, the canula should be pushed still further in. The surgeon should be ready at once to close the canula with his thumb, if the flow begins to cease, lest air should be admitted. If the flow ceases from any cause before all the fluid seems to be evacuated, the trocar should not be re-introduced, lest the intestines be wounded, but a blunt-headed perforated instrument fitting the canula should be inserted.

When all the fluid that can be easily obtained is evacuated, the canula may be withdrawn, and a pad of lint secured over the wound by strapping.

GASTROTOMY.—Cutting into the stomach for the extraction of a foreign body has now been performed at least ten times, and all but one recovered. A typical example is that by Dr. Bell of Davenport, who removed a bar of lead one pound in weight and ten inches in length, by an incision four inches in length from the umbilicus to the false ribs. The opening into the stomach was as small as possible, and required no sutures.

GASTROSTOMY has within the last few years been practised very frequently. Gross has collected 79 cases, 57 of which were for carcinoma of œsophagus, all of which died within a few weeks, except eight who survived for periods varying from three to seven months. The results in cases of cicatricial and syphilitic strictures are more favourable.—Howse's method seems the best, consisting of two stages.

1. A curved incision is made through the parietes parallel with, and a finger-breadth below, the lower margin of chest wall on left side, the peritoneum should be opened at the linea semilunaris, the stomach sought for, and then attached to the abdominal wall by an outer ring of sutures and to the edge of the wound by an inner ring. It should then be dressed with carbolised lint and supported by a bandage.

2. A small opening should be made four or five days after the first stage and the patient should be fed through this opening.

For full details, see Mr. Durham's paper in vol. i. of Holmes's Surgery, edition of 1883, pp. 801-4.

GASTRECTOMY.—Excision of whole or part of the stomach is one of the latest developments of operative daring, first done as a regular operation by Pean in 1879, it has now been repeated sixteen times; four cases have survived the operation for more than ten days. The chief points to be attended to are prevention of death from shock and hæmorrhage, and very careful stitching up of the wound. Considering the difficulty of the diagnosis, the danger of the operation, and the almost certain recurrence of the disease, the propriety of such operation seems very doubtful.

OVARIOTOMY.—For the pathology of ovarian disease we must refer to Sir Spencer Wells's work on the subject, and to the smaller Monograph on Ovarian Pathology, by the late lamented Dr. Charles Ritchie, junior.

Even the modifications in the method of operating which have been devised are so various and numerous, that if collected from the medical journals of the last ten years they would fill a large volume. Besides this, the operation of ovariotomy is one attended by so many complications, that individual cases vary from each other as much as do individual cases of hernia and tracheotomy; and as the specialities of each case require to be met by specialities of treatment, there is hardly any operation in surgery which requires greater readiness of invention, or more individual sagacity in the operator.

To lay open the abdominal cavity from the sternum to the pubes, and rapidly dissect out of this cavity an enormous tumour with a narrow neck, the operator's only embarrassment being the peristaltic movements of the bowels, and his only care being to tie the neck of the tumour firmly with strong string, sew up the wound, and trust to nature, was an operation very easy to perform, and requiring free cutting rather than dexterity, and rashness more than true surgical insight.

Such were the ovariotomies prior to 1857.

An ovariotomy in 1883 is a very different business, varying in certain important particulars.

(1.) Instead of the incision extending from sternum to pubes, it is now made as short as possible.

(2.) Instead of being removed entire, the cyst is now emptied with the greatest possible care (prior to its removal), and none of the contents allowed to enter the peritoneal cavity.

(3.) The pedicle is brought to the surface, and in every case where it is possible is secured outside the wound.

Besides these three important and cardinal points, there are other minor matters almost equally essential; these are—(1.) The proper management of the adhesions and the thorough prevention of all hæmorrhage from them; (2.) the stitching up of the external wound, including the peritoneum; (3.) the treatment of the patient during the first few days of convalescence.

Operation in a typical case, after the method of Sir Spencer Wells and Dr. Thomas Keith.—The patient having had her bowels gently opened on the previous day, and being as far as possible in her usual state of health, should be warmly clad in flannel, both in body and limb, and laid on an operating table of convenient height, in or near the room she is to occupy. No carrying from ward to operating theatre and back again is admissible. It will be found both cleanly and convenient to have a large india-rubber cloth over the whole abdomen, cut out in the centre so as to expose so much of the tumour as is necessary, but gummed on or otherwise secured to the sides of the abdomen, and thus protecting the clothes, and hanging down over the edge of the table; this will prevent all wetting of the clothes and unnecessary exposure of the patient's person, and can be easily removed after the operation. Chloroform being administered, the bladder is evacuated by means of a catheter, and the patient's head and shoulders are elevated on pillows. An incision is then made in the linea alba, between the umbilicus and pubes, for about four inches in length at first, so as to be large enough to admit the hand, through all the tissues down to and through the peritoneum. Care is necessary in dividing the peritoneum, on the one hand, not to divide too much, in which case the cyst-wall will be penetrated, and the contents effused into the peritoneal cavity; or, on the other hand, too little, in which case the peritoneum may be mistaken for the cyst, and separated from the transversalis fascia under the idea that adhesions exist. Once the peritoneal cavity is opened, the incision through the peritoneum must be extended to the full length of the external wound by a probe-pointed bistoury.

The operator's hand must now be passed into the abdomen, and the tumour isolated from its connections as far as possible. When no adhesions exist it is extremely easy to pass the hand quite round the tumour, ascertain its relations to the uterus and Fallopian tubes, and the length and thickness of its pedicle. The presence of adhesions adds very seriously to the danger and duration of the operation. We will suppose at present that none exist in this typical case, and that the pedicle is found of a satisfactory size and shape. The surgeon now protrudes the anterior portion of the cyst-wall through the wound, and pierces it with a large trocar,[139] to which is attached an india-rubber tube, by means of which the effused fluid can be easily got rid of in any direction. During the escape of the fluid from the cyst a special assistant keeps up the tension by careful pressure on the abdomen. In cases where the cyst is multilocular, and thus only a portion of the contents of the tumour is at first evaluated, the operator should, by partially withdrawing the trocar, without removing it entirely from the cyst, endeavour to pierce and evacuate the other cysts, still through the original opening in the first one.

While doing this, great care must be taken lest he pierce the external wall of the tumour, and let any of the contents escape into the abdominal cavity; to guard against this, the punctures should be made by the right hand, while the left, re-inserted into the abdomen, supports the cyst-wall.

The tumour having been as far as possible emptied of its fluid contents, must now be dragged out of the wound, care being still taken lest any of its fluid contents escape into the peritoneal cavity. In favourable cases the pedicle is now brought easily into view. This may vary very much in length and thickness. It is sometimes entirely absent,

---

[139] Description of Sir Spencer Wells's Trocar.—"It consists of a hollow cylinder six inches long, and half an inch in diameter, within which another cylinder fitting it tightly plays. The inner one is cut off at its extremity, somewhat in the form of a pen, and is sharp. The sharp end is kept retracted within the outer cylinder by a spiral spring in the handle at the other end, but can be protruded by pressing on this handle when required for use. When thus protruded it is plunged into the cyst up to its middle; the pressure on the handle is taken off, and the cutting edge is retracted within its sheath. The fluid rushes into the tube, and escapes by an aperture in the side, to which an india-rubber tube is attached, the end of which drops into a bucket under the table. The instrument is furnished at its middle with two semicircular bars, carrying each four or five long curved teeth like a vulsellum. These teeth lie in contact with the outer surface of the cylinder, but can be raised from it by pressing two handles. When the cyst begins to be flaccid by the escape of the fluid, these side vulsellums are raised, and the adjoining part of the cyst is drawn up under the teeth, where it is firmly caught and compressed against the side of the tube."

the tumour being sessile on the broad ligament of the uterus; sometimes it is thick and strong, sometimes long and slender. The manner in which it is to be managed depends on its length and thickness. Varieties in treatment will be noticed immediately. We will suppose that it is four inches in length and one or two fingers in breadth. This is quite a suitable case for the use of the clamp, the principle involved in the use of which is, that the pedicle should be brought quite out of the abdomen through the wound and secured on the surface. The best form seems to be one made like a carpenter's callipers, with long but removable handles, and a very powerful fixing-screw.

The blades of this clamp being protected by pads of lint should be made to embrace the pedicle close to the cyst, in a direction at right angles to the abdominal wound, and lying across it, the handles should then be removed, and pads of lint placed below the clamp to protect the skin. The cyst may now be cut away at some little distance above the clamp, enough being left to prevent all danger of its slipping. Further to avoid this danger, the pedicle may be transfixed by one or two needles above the clamp.

The wound is now to be sewed up by several points of interrupted suture, some inserted very deeply through all the tissues, including even the peritoneum, others in the intervals of the first, including little more than the skin. They may be either of iron, silver, platinum, telegraph-wire (Mr. Clover's copper, coated with gutta-percha), or silk. It seems of very little consequence which is used. Sir Spencer Wells, after many trials, uses silk, as being removed with least pain to the patient, and really causing no more suppuration than the metallic ones do, if only removed early enough, viz., about the second or third day, by which time the union of the wound should be firm.

The after-treatment should be very simple. Except under special circumstances, stimulants are rarely necessary, and indeed, to avoid vomiting, as little as possible should be given by the mouth during the first twenty-four hours. The patient should be allowed to suck a little ice to allay thirst, and opiate and nutritive enemata will be found quite sufficient to keep up the strength in ordinary cases. The urine should be drawn off by the catheter every six hours. The room should be kept quiet, and the temperature equable, so long as there is no interference with a plentiful supply of fresh air.

Some of the specialities and abnormalities involving special risks may now be briefly noticed:—

1. *Adhesions.*—These vary much in amount, in position, in organisation, and danger.

a. *In amount.*—In certain cases no adhesions exist, while in others, omentum, intestines, tumour, uterus, and abdominal wall may be all matted together in one common mass.

b. *In organisation.*—Occasionally they are so soft and friable as

160

to break down under the finger with ease, and so slightly organised as not to bleed at all in the process, while again they may be so firm and close as to require a careful and prolonged dissection, and so vascular as to require many points of ligature to be applied to large active vessels.

c. There are special dangers connected with the presence of these adhesions, and varying much in different cases. Thus adhesions to the intestines can generally be separated with comparative ease, and seem, as a rule, to require the application of fewer ligatures than those which unite the tumour to the abdominal wall. Adhesions to the wall are sometimes so firm as to be quite inseparable, and thus to necessitate some of the cyst-wall being left adherent. In Sir Spencer Wells's cases, adhesions to the liver and gall-bladder occasionally occurred, requiring careful dissection to separate them, and yet the patients all survived, while pelvic adhesions, especially to the bladder and uterus, on more than one occasion prevented the completion of the operation.

Vascular adhesions to the wall which require many ligatures certainly add to the dangers of the case, while adhesions to the anterior wall of the abdomen render the operation, especially its first stages, much more difficult, preventing the cyst from being recognised.

2. *The condition of the pedicle* is of great importance. If it is too short, it prevents the use of the clamp, as if applied it is apt either to pull the uterus up, or, pulling the clamp down, to make undue traction on the wound, and rupture any adhesions. This is especially the case where much flatus is generated, or where the patient is naturally stout.

Treatment.—Where the pedicle is just long enough to allow the clamp to be applied, and yet too short to leave room for any distension of the abdomen without undue tension, the best plan is to transfix it with a stout double thread just below the clamp, tie it in two halves, and bring the threads out past the clamp, so that, if tension does occur, the clamp may be removed, the part beyond it cut off, and the rest allowed to slip back into the pelvis, the ligatures being kept out at the mouth of the wound.

Or again, it is sometimes possible, after applying one clamp firmly as near the tumour as possible, to apply another above it when the greater part of the tumour has been cut away; when the second is firmly fixed it may then be safe to remove the first, and thus an artificially elongated pedicle is obtained.

When still shorter, two plans remain for selection—(1.) to transfix the pedicle in one or more points, then, securing it in two, three, or more portions, cut it off above the ligatures and return it, leaving the ligatures at the lower end of the wound. This gives a free drain for pus, but theoretically the sloughing pedicle might be expected to set up peritonitis; (2.) to transfix and tie the pedicle with one or more loops of stout string, cut the ends off short, and return the whole affair, closing the external wound at once. Theoretically there are grave

161

objections to this plan, but it has proved very successful, especially in the hands of Dr. Tyler Smith.

Another ingenious modification, sometimes useful in a short narrow pedicle, is to tie it as close to the cyst as possible, bring the ligature out at the wound, and then with a strong harelip needle transfix the pedicle, along with both sides of the wound, just below the ligature.

When the pedicle is excessively broad and stout, it should be transfixed by strong needles and double threads in various places, and thus tied in several portions. Absence of the pedicle greatly adds to the danger in any given case. Various plans have been tried, as cutting the attachment through slowly by the écraseur, ligature of each vessel separately, so many as twelve being sometimes required, and cauterising the stump. The latter, as used by Mr. Baker Brown, has met with a large measure of success, and is much used now.[140]

Dr. Keith for a time operated with antiseptic precautions, but has now (1883) entirely given up the use of the spray, which he believes has especial dangers in abdominal surgery.

OPERATION FOR STRANGULATED INGUINAL HERNIA.— The great rule to be remembered with regard to this, as well as all other operations for hernia, is, that the earlier it is performed the better chance the patient has. Once a fair trial has been given to the taxis, aided by proper position of the patient, the warm bath, and specially chloroform, the operation should be performed.

The patient should be placed on his back with his shoulders elevated, and the knee of the affected side slightly bent. The groin should then be shaved, and the shape and size of the tumour, with the position of the inguinal canal, carefully studied. The surgeon should then lift up a fold of skin and cellular tissue, in a direction at right angles to the long axis of the tumour, and holding one side of this raised fold in his own left hand, commit the other to an assistant. He then transfixes this fold with a sharp straight bistoury, with its back towards the sac, and cuts outwards, thus at once making an incision along the axis of the hernia without any risk of wounding the sac or bowel. Any vessel that bleeds may now be tied. This incision will be found sufficiently large for most cases; if not, however, it can easily be prolonged either upwards or downwards. The surgeon must now devote his attention to exposing the neck of the sac, and in so doing, defining the external inguinal ring. The safest method of doing so is carefully to pinch up, with dissecting forceps, layer after layer of

---

[140] For further details on the operations described above, reference may be made to Sir Spencer Wells's work on ovarian disease, and to the very valuable papers contributed by Dr. Thomas Keith to the Edinburgh Medical Journal. To the latter especially the author is indebted for much oral instruction, and for the opportunity of seeing his careful and dexterous mode of operating.

connective tissue, dividing each separately by the knife held with its flat side, not its edge, on the sac, and then by means of the finger or forceps raising each layer in succession and dividing it to the full extent of the external incision. It is not always an easy matter to recognise the sac, especially as the number of layers above it, which are described in the anatomical text-books, are often not at all distinct.

The thickness of the connective tissue of the part varies immensely; sometimes six layers or even more can be separately dissected, while, again, one only may be found before the sac is exposed.

If small and recent, the sac may be recognised by its bluish colour, and by the fact that it is possible to pinch up a portion of it between the finger and thumb, and thus to rub its opposed surfaces against each other.

If large and of old standing, it is sometimes so thin as not to be recognisable, or again so enormously thickened, and so adherent, as to be defined with great difficulty.

If it is small, i.e. when the whole tumour is under the size of an egg, it ought to be thoroughly isolated, and its boundaries everywhere defined. If large, and specially if adherent, the neck alone should be cleared.

The sac thus being reached, the external abdominal ring should be clearly defined, and the finger passed into it so as if possible to determine the presence or absence of any constriction in it. If it feels tight, the internal pillar of the ring should then be cautiously divided on the finger by a probe-pointed narrow bistoury, in a direction parallel to the linea alba.

At this stage the question comes to be considered as to whether the sac should or should not be opened. Much has been said and written on both sides.

Not to open the sac avoids the risk of peritonitis, and of injury to the bowel; but, on the other hand, exposes the patient to the danger of the hernia being returned unreduced; for in many cases the stricture is to be found in the sac itself, and adhesions very rapidly form between coils of intestine in the sac and the inner wall. Again, not to open the sac prevents us from discovering the condition in which the bowel is; it may possibly be gangrenous, in which case such a return en masse would be almost necessarily fatal.

A general rule or two may be given here:—

1. The sac should be opened in every case where there is any reason for doubt about the condition of the bowel, where there has been long-continued vomiting, or much tenderness on pressure.

2. Even in cases in which there is every reason to believe the bowel is perfectly sound, the sac should be opened, unless the whole contents can be easily and completely reduced out of the sac into the belly, as in cases where this cannot be done there probably exist either

a stricture in the neck of the sac itself, or adhesions of the bowel to the sac. We should endeavour to avoid opening the sac in cases of old scrotal hernia of large size, where the symptoms have not been urgent, especially in large unhealthy hospitals, as the risk of peritonitis is so great. Antiseptic precautions seem considerably to diminish the risk of opening the sac.

If the sac then is not to be opened, the rest of the operation is very simple. Endeavour to reduce the bowel out of the sac, and then return the sac itself, unless the hernia is of old standing, and adhesions prevent its reduction. A few silver stitches to close the wound and a carefully adjusted pad are now all that is requisite.

If the sac is to be opened, how can it be done with least danger to the bowel?

If the hernia is small, and it is possible to define it all, the sac should be opened at its lower end, as there a small quantity of serous fluid which intervenes between the sac and the bowel will be found. Where this is present, there is no danger of wounding the bowel, as the sac can be easily pinched up; but this is by no means invariably the case, so great care should always be taken. A small portion of the wall being thus pinched up should be divided in the same manner as the layers of cellular tissue were divided in exposing the sac. A few drops of serum will then escape, and the glistening surface of the bowel be exposed; the finger should then be introduced at the opening, and the incision enlarged by a probe-pointed bistoury. If the hernia is small the sac should be slit up to its full extent; if large, only a sufficient portion of the neck should be opened. As soon as the opening in the sac is large enough to admit the point of the operator's forefinger, it should be inserted so as to protect the intestines, and the remainder of the sac slit up on it as a guide.

The sac thus opened, the next step is to divide the constriction, wherever it be. It is most likely to be found at the neck of the sac, just where it protrudes through the internal ring in an oblique hernia, or through the tendons of the transversalis and internal oblique, where the hernia is direct. Now, this constriction might be divided in any direction were it not for the risk of wounding the epigastric artery, and also of injuring the spermatic cord, which is in close relation to the neck of the sac of an oblique hernia.

Wound of the epigastric artery is the chief danger, for in all cases it is close to the neck of the sac. Were its position in relation to the neck of the sac constant, it might be easily avoided by an incision in the opposite direction; but as this relation varies according to the nature of the hernia, an element of danger is introduced. Thus, in oblique inguinal ruptures, where the sac passes out through the internal ring (Fig. xxxii. ir), the artery will always be found to the inside of the neck of the sac; while in direct herniæ, where the bowel has made its escape through the triangle of Hesselbach (Fig. xxxii. +), and passed through the conjoint tendon straight to the external ring, the epigastric artery will be found on the outside of the neck of the sac. In recent herniæ the differential diagnosis is comparatively easy, but in those of old standing and large size, in which the obliquity of the canal has been much diminished, it is almost impossible to tell of what kind the hernia originally was, and consequently to determine in which direction it is safe to incise the neck of the sac.

Such being the case, the best rule is to incise the neck of the sac directly upwards, i.e. in a line parallel with the linea alba, and also to cut it very cautiously bit by bit, in every case, if possible, with the finger inserted as a guide to the position of a vessel and a protection to the gut.

The spermatic vessels lie sometimes behind, sometimes on either side of the sac, and in very old herniæ may be separated from each other so as really to surround the sac. The cut directly upwards is also the safest for them.

All constrictions being overcome, it is not sufficient merely to push back the gut into the belly. Its condition must be carefully examined, and it must be decided whether the constriction has caused gangrene or not. To examine this properly, it is generally best to pull down an inch or two more of the gut, so as thoroughly to bring into view the constricted portion, as it is most likely to be fatally nipped.

It is not always easy to decide as to the condition of the bowel. Certain points must be observed:—

(1.) *Colour.*—There may be very great alteration in the colour of the bowel from congestion, and yet no gangrene. It may be dark red, claret, purple, or even have a brownish tint, and yet recover; where it is black, or a deep brown, the prognosis is unfavourable.

(2.) *Glistening.*—So long as the proper glistening appearance of the bowel remains, there is hope for it, even when the colour is bad; if it has lost it, and especially if, instead of being tense and shining, it is dull and flaccid and in wrinkles, the bowel is almost certainly gangrenous.

(3.) *Thickness.*—If much thickened, and especially if rough on the surface, the bowel has probably been forming adhesions to the sac, or to contiguous coils, and the prognosis is less favourable.

(4.) *Smell.*—The peculiar gangrenous odour on opening the sac is very characteristic. In cases where ulceration and perforation have occurred, the odour is fæcal.

1. If, then, the bowel is tolerably healthy-looking, though discoloured, it should be returned gradually, not en masse, into the abdomen, the wound sewed up, and a pad of lint put on, with a bandage.

2. If there are adhesions of bowel to sac or to a neighbouring coil, or of omentum to sac, the stricture should be freely divided, the protruding coils of intestine should be emptied of their contents, but no rash attempt made to force their return. Especially is this rule to be

observed with protruded, swollen, or adherent omentum, for considerable risks attend any attempt at excision of the protruded portion—risks of hæmorrhage, peritonitis, and ulceration of the contiguous bowel.

If the bowel be returned, or even the continuity of the canal restored by the cutting of the stricture, though the bowel be not returned, no great risks accrue from the retention of a piece of omentum in the sac, in a position which it may possibly have already occupied for years.

3. If the bowel is absolutely gangrenous, even in a very small portion of its length, no reduction should be attempted, but the gangrenous portion should be kept outside, with the hope that adhesive inflammation may be set up, so as to glue the bowel to the abdominal wall, prevent fæcal extravasation, and form a temporary artificial anus. If the gangrenous portion be very full of fæces or flatus, incisions may be made into it. This should be avoided in cases where the patient is already much prostrated, as I have seen cases in which the opening of the bowel seemed to inflict a fatal shock.

Enterectomy or excision of the gangrenous portion has recently been recommended and performed by some surgeons. The very high authority of the late Professor Spence is against such procedure.[141]

Cases of gangrene of even large portions of bowel are by no means necessarily fatal. They may recover with an artificial anus, the remedy of which by surgical means we must notice in its proper place.

OPERATION FOR STRANGULATED FEMORAL HERNIA.— While the general principles guiding treatment and ruling the conduct of the operation are the same as in inguinal, there are some differences in points of detail which render a brief separate description necessary.

A single word on the anatomy. Tracing a femoral rupture from within outwards, we find that its first stage is to push its way through the weak point of the arch formed by Poupart's ligament, that is, the spot called the crural arch, bounded on its outer side by the sheath of fascia which surrounds the femoral vein; above by Poupart's ligament; on its inner side by the curved fibres of Poupart's ligament, which, curving backwards, are inserted into the ilio-pectineal line, have a sharp falciform edge, and have been dignified by the special name of Gimbernat's ligament (Fig. xxxii. g); and below by the os pubis itself. This arch or ring thus bounded is, in the normal state of parts, filled by a layer of fibrous texture, a little fat, and occasionally a small gland. These parts are pushed forwards in the descent of the hernia, and in a small recent one may be said to form a sort of inner covering; in a larger and older one they are split by the hernia, and, while forming a constriction round its neck, leave

---

[141] Lect. on Surgery, 3d ed., vol. ii. p. 998.

the fundus of the sac, so far as they are concerned, quite uncovered.

A femoral hernia may stop there, satisfied with merely coming through the ring, and, if sudden and recent in a healthy, well-knit subject, such a rupture is exceedingly dangerous, the constriction being very severe, and the consequent gangrene of the bowel very rapid if unrelieved. In most cases, however, it makes its way still further out, and the next covering it gains is from the cribriform fascia. This is the layer of fibres, pierced (as its name implies) with orifices for the passage of veins and lymphatics, which stretches between the two curved edges of the saphenous opening. It varies much in strength; when the rupture has been slow and gradual, it will certainly add a covering of greater or less thickness, but where the hernia is large and old we must not expect to find many traces of the cribriform fascia, at least over the fundus of the tumour.

The ordinary superficial fascia of the part, with its fat, nerves, veins, and lymphatics, and the thin skin of the groin, are the only remaining coverings. It is very remarkable how exceedingly thin all the so-called coats become in large femoral herniæ of long standing, especially in thin old people.

Operation.—Various incisions are recommended. The one which gives freest access and exposes the sac best, is shaped like a T, the horizontal limb of which is oblique, the direction of the obliquity varying on the two sides. The horizontal incision should be made just over Poupart's ligament, and parallel to it, the centre of the incision corresponding to the neck of the sac, and its length varying according to the size of the tumour and the depth of the parts; the other should extend downwards from the centre of the former, as far as is necessary to display the whole sac. The first should be made by pinching up and transfixing the skin, the second by ordinary incision, to the same depth as the first. The small flaps thus made must now be thrown back; any vessels that have been divided are to be tied. Now, with great care and caution the surgeon is to pinch up and divide any layers of condensed cellular tissue which may still cover the sac, till it is thoroughly exposed to its full extent, and remove any glands which may intervene.

The neck of the sac being exposed, it may be possible in some very exceptional cases to give the patient the benefit of the minor operation, which consists in leaving the sac unopened. In such a case (to be described immediately), the surgeon passes his finger along the neck of the sac as far as possible into the ring, and then with a probe-pointed bistoury very cautiously nicks the upper edge of Gimbernat's ligament, in one or more places, being careful to feel for any pulsation before dividing a single fibre. He may then be able to empty the sac of its contents, and return the bowel and omentum, still retaining the sac outside.

On the other hand, where it is determined to open the sac, the

167

pinching up of the sac must be managed with great care, to avoid injury of the bowel. There is generally a little fluid to be found at the fundus, which will protect the bowel. In one case in which Liston operated, he tells us, "there was no possibility of pinching up the sac, either with the fingers or forceps; it contained no fluid, and was impacted most firmly with bowel; very luckily the membrane was thin; and, observing a pelleton of fat underneath, I scratched very cautiously with the point of the knife in the unsupported hand, until a trifling puncture was made, sufficient to admit the blunt point of a narrow bistoury."[142] If the sac contains bowel and omentum, it is safer to open it over the omentum than over the bowel. When a small opening is made, an escape of the contained fluid takes place, and then the sac should be slit up as far as its neck by a probe-pointed bistoury, guided by the finger, introduced to protect the bowel, whenever the opening is sufficiently large. The forefinger must now be cautiously insinuated into the neck of the sac, the nail being directed to the bowel, the pulp to the crescentic margin of Gimbernat's ligament, and any constriction very cautiously divided. The bowel should then be drawn down a little, the constricted point carefully examined, and then returned or not, according to its condition.

Two points require a brief separate notice:—

1. In what direction is the crural arch to be divided? Not outwards certainly, on account of the vein, nor downwards, as the bone prevents that direction. Is it to be upwards or inwards? Not upwards, for such an incision would endanger the spermatic cord or round ligament, besides greatly weakening the abdominal wall by the division, partial or complete, of Poupart's ligament. Inwards then it must be; and little more need be said about it, were it not for the occasional existence of an abnormal course and distribution of the obturator artery.

Fig.xxxii.[143]

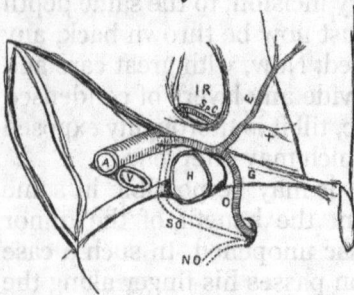

The usual origin of this vessel is from the internal iliac, in which case (Fig. xxxii. n o) it never comes near the sac at all. In certain cases (1 in 3½) it rises from the epigastric, and in a very few (1 in 72) from the external iliac. If rising from either of the two last, it

---

142 Operative Surgery, p. 462.
143 Rough diagram of abnormal course of obturator and its relation to the neck of a hernia. Parts seen from the inside: h, femoral hernia; a, femoral artery; v, femoral vein; e, epigastric artery; o, obturator from epigastric (dangerous); s o, obturator from epigastric (safe); n o, normal course of obturator; i r, internal inguinal ring; Sp c, spermatic chord and its vessels; g, Gimbernat's ligament; +, in triangle of Hesselbach.

most commonly passes downwards at the outer side of the hernia, in which case (Fig. xxxii. s o) no harm can possibly result; but in a few rare cases, perhaps 1 in every 60 of those operated on, the vessel winds round the hernia (Fig. xxxii. o), crossing at its inner side, and thus may be (and has actually been) divided by a rash incision. With due care, however, and by cutting a very little at a time, even this danger may be avoided.

2. Under what circumstances is it possible or justifiable to reduce a femoral hernia, without previously opening the sac? Only in certain very select cases, where the hernia is recent, the constricting parts lax, the general symptoms very mild, and where there is reason to believe the bowel has completely escaped injury by compression or the taxis. There are both difficulties and dangers in this so-called minor operation:—1. Difficulties, For it is not easy to divide the constriction without the assistance of the finger in the sac, and it is not easy to reduce the contents with the sac unopened, except through a much freer opening than is necessary when the bowel has been fairly exposed. 2. Dangers, Of reducing sac and viscera, together with the strangulation still kept up by tightness in the neck of the sac; or of supposing the sac is emptied while a knuckle of bowel still remains in it, and is strangulated; or, lastly, of reducing the intestine which has already become gangrenous. It is very remarkable how very soon gangrene may come on, in a case of a small recent femoral hernia, in which the fibrous tissues constricting the neck of the sac are tense and undilatable. A protrusion for eight hours has been sufficient to destroy the life of a knuckle of bowel.

A note here on a certain condition very frequent in femoral herniæ, which may occasionally give a good deal of trouble. Symptoms of strangulation have been well marked, yet when the sac is opened nothing is to be seen except a mass of omentum, perhaps tolerably healthy-looking. To reduce this en masse would be very unsafe; it is necessary carefully to unravel it, and disengage the knuckle of bowel which is almost certainly included in it, and which has given rise to the symptoms of strangulation.

OPERATION FOR STRANGULATED UMBILICAL HERNIA.— The operation is practically the same, whether the hernia is a true umbilical one, or one which with more strict accuracy might be called ventral. True umbilical hernia is a disease of infancy and childhood, being almost always congenital, and the viscera protrude through the umbilical aperture. This rarely requires operation, as it may generally be returned with ease, and even cured by a proper bandage and compress. Ventral hernia, commonly called umbilical, is generally a protrusion of viscera through a new preternatural aperture in the fibrous tissues close to the navel, may often attain a large size, is liable to strangulation, and is not easily palliated or cured.

In either case the operation requires a very brief description. If the hernia is small, under the size of a hen's egg, a crucial incision through the thin skin which covers it will thoroughly expose the sac when the flaps are dissected back. The forefinger should then be inserted in the round opening, and the edges cautiously incised in several directions, each incision however being very small.

If the rupture is large, a single linear, or a T-shaped incision, exposing the base of the tumour, will be sufficient to allow the requisite dilatation of the opening to be made. It is not at all necessary in every case to open the sac of the peritoneum. If required, it must be done with great caution, as the sac is generally very thin. In cases where the hernia is chiefly omental, the sac should be opened, lest a knuckle of bowel be inclosed and strangulated in the omentum.

Obturator Hernia is an extremely rare lesion, and a large proportion of the recorded cases were discovered only after death. When diagnosed during life and strangulated, some have been reduced by taxis, and only a very few cases have been operated on, some with success. It is not likely that a diagnosis could be made, except in very emaciated patients, in whom pain at the obturator foramen was a prominent symptom, and in whom it could be ascertained positively that the crural ring was empty. An incision over the tumour, sufficient to allow the pectineus muscle to be exposed and divided, is necessary. The hernia may then be reduced without opening the sac, if recent; if of long standing, the sac must be opened. One case is recorded by Dr. Lorinzer, in which, after strangulation for eleven days, he opened the sac and found the bowel gangrenous. The patient had a fæcal fistula; but survived the operation for eleven months. Nuttel, Obrè, and Bransby Cooper have each diagnosed and treated such cases.[144]

Other forms of hernia are so rare, and the treatment of each case must necessarily vary so much in its circumstances, as not to require or admit of any detailed account of the operations requisite for their relief.

OPERATIONS FOR THE RADICAL CURE OF HERNIA.—The inconveniences and discomfort caused by even the best-adjusted trusses or bandages, the unsatisfactory support they afford, and the risk of their slipping and allowing the hernia to escape, have given rise to many attempts to cure hernia by operation.

Even to enumerate these would be quite beyond the limits of the present volume; suffice it to classify a few of the most important of them according to the principle involved in each, and then give a very brief account of the method of operating which seems to be at once the most scientific, least dangerous, and most permanently useful.

The question at issue is briefly this. We have, in a hernia, the following condition:—The walls of a great cavity are at one or more points specially weak, the contained viscera have protruded, either by

144 Holmes's Surgery, 3d ed., 1883, vol. ii. p. 837.

extension and stretching of a natural opening, or by the formation of a new breach in the walls, and, in protruding, they have brought with them as a covering a serous membrane, extremely extensible, highly sensitive to injury, and, when injured, certain to resent it by severe, spreading, and dangerous inflammation.

Do we desire to remedy this protrusion, we may act—

1. On the intestines themselves; but for all surgical purposes, they are out of our reach. We cannot do more than, by diminishing their contents, diminish their volume, and by position and rest reduce to the utmost their tendency to protrude. This includes the medical and prophylactic treatment of hernia, or rather of the tendency to hernia.

2. We may try what can be done with the sac which the intestines have pushed down before them. Can it be obliterated? If it can, perhaps the intestines may be retained in their cavity. Very many plans of dealing with the sac have been tried.

To cause obliteration of its cavity many methods have been proposed:—by ligature of it along with the spermatic cord, involving loss of the testicle, either by gradual separation, by sloughing, or by immediate removal;—by cutting into it, and then stitching it up;—by constricting it with wire, as in the punctum aureum; by pinching sac and coverings up, by passing needles under them as they emerge from the external ring, as Bonnet of Lyons did; by constricting sac alone with a double wire, by subcutaneous puncture, as Dr. Morton of Glasgow has done;—by severe pressure from the outside with a strong tight truss and a pad of wood, as proposed by Richter; by setons of threads or candlewicks, as proposed by Schuh of Vienna;—by injection of tincture of iodine or cantharides, as by Velpeau and Pancoast;—by the introduction into the sac of thin bladders of goldbeaters' skin, which were then filled with air, and were intended to excite inflammation, as in the radical cure of hydrocele; or by the still more severe method of Langenbeck, consisting in exposing the sac by a free incision at the superficial ring, separating it from the cord, and passing a ligature round the sac alone, leaving the ligatured portion in the scrotum either to become obliterated or to slough out. Schmucker of Berlin varied this, by cutting away the constricted portion below the ligature.

The objections to these methods are various: the more gentle are uncertain and inefficient; of the more severe, some involve mutilation, by the loss or removal of the testicle; others, as those of Langenbeck and Schmucker, are very dangerous and fatal, by the inflammation spreading to the peritoneal cavity (20 to 30 per cent. died); while all of these methods afford at best only temporary relief. And this is only what might have been expected, for the sac was only a result of the protrusion, not a cause; and so long as the weakness and insufficiency of the parietes of the abdomen remain, so long will the extensible loosely-attached peritoneum continue to furnish new sacs for visceral protrusions.

3. We have now only the canal left to act upon; and the operations on the canal may be divided into two great classes:—

(a.) Those in which the operator attempts to plug up the dilated canal. (b.) Those in which he tries to constrict it, by reuniting its separated sides.

(a.) Attempts to plug the canal have, in most cases, been made by invagination of the skin of the scrotum and its fascia. These have been very numerous and various in their adaptation of mechanical appliances, but have all been designed with the same object. Dzondi of Halle, and Jameson of Baltimore, incised lancet-shaped flaps of skin, and endeavoured to fix them by displacement over the ring. Gerdy invaginated a portion of scrotum and fascia into the enlarged canal, by the forefinger pushed it up, and secured it in its place by a thread passed from the point of his finger first through the invaginated skin, then through the abdominal walls, endeavouring to include the walls of the inguinal canal, causing the point of the needle to project some lines above the inguinal ring; the same process being effected with the other end of the thread on the other side of the finger, and the two ends which have been brought out near each other on the abdominal wall, being tied tightly over a cylinder of plaster. The ensheathed sac was then painted with caustic ammonia to excite inflammation, and a pad put on over all.

Signoroni modified this by fixing the invaginated skin by a piece of female catheter, retained in its place by transfixion by three harelip needles, tied by twisted sutures.

Wützer of Bonn, again, modified this, by substituting a complicated instrument, consisting of a stout plug in the inguinal canal, held in position by needles which are passed through the anterior wall of the canal in the groin. Compression between plug and compress, with the intention of causing adhesion between skin, fascia, and sac, is then managed by means of a screw. The plug is retained for about seven days.

Modifications of this method have been tried by Wells, Rothmund, and Redfern Davies, all aiming in the direction of simplicity; but by far the most simple and efficacious method on the Wützer principle yet devised is that of Professor Syme, which he described in the pages of the Edinburgh Medical Journal for May 1861, in which the invagination of integument is both simply and securely managed by strong threads, as in Gerdy's method, while a piece of bougie or gutta-percha, to which the threads are fixed, replaces Wützer's expensive and complicated apparatus. Sir J. Fayrer of Calcutta has had a very large experience of Wützer's method, and also of a plan of his own. Out of 102 cases by the latter method, 77 were cured, 9 relieved, 14 failed, and 2 died.[145]

---

[145] Clinical and Pathological Observations in India, pp. 44, 325.

Mr. Pritchard of Bristol has proposed an additional step in operations on the invagination principle, consisting in the stripping of a thin slip of skin from the orifice of the cutaneous canal, and then putting a pin through the parts to get them to unite, and thus close the aperture completely.

Now, what results follow these operations? At first they are almost invariably successful, but the complaint is that, in most cases, the rupture recurs. The principle is to plug up the passage by the mechanical presence of the invaginated skin, the plug being retained in position by adhesive inflammation between it and the edges of the dilated ring. But the ring is left dilated, or, indeed, generally its dilatation is increased; and as, on continued pressure from within, the new adhesions give way, or, as often happens, a new protrusion takes place in the circular cul-de-sac necessarily left all round the apex of the invagination, the still lax ring and canal offer no resistance to the protrusion.

(b.) The principle of constriction of the canal by reuniting its separated sides. This is the principle of the various methods introduced by Mr. Wood of King's College, and described by him in his most able and exhaustive work.[146]

He applies sutures through the sides of the dilated inguinal or crural canals, or umbilical openings, in such a manner as to insure their complete closure.

1. For inguinal hernia.—To stitch together the two sides of the canal with safety requires attention to several points—(1.) That it be done nearly, if not entirely, subcutaneously. (2.) That the protruding bowel should be kept out of the way, and not be transfixed by the needle. (3.) That the spermatic cord should be protected from injurious pressure.

These different indications are attained by Mr. Wood by a very ingenious mode of operating, which I can describe here only briefly, and for a full description of which I must refer to Mr. Wood's own monograph already alluded to.

For his first twenty cases Mr. Wood used strong hempen thread for the stitches; of late, however, he has proved the greater advantage of strong wire.

When a large old hernia in an adult is the subject of operation, it is thus performed by Mr. Wood:—The pubes being shaved, and the patient put thoroughly under the influence of chloroform, the rupture is reduced, and the operator's forefinger forced up the canal so as to push every morsel of bowel fairly into the abdomen. An assistant then commands the internal ring by pressure, to prevent return of the rupture.

An incision is made in the scrotum over the fundus of the sac,

---

[146] Wood On Rupture, 1863.

large enough to admit a forefinger and the large needle used in the operation; the edges of the skin are to be separated from the fascia below for about one inch all round. The forefinger is then to be passed in at the aperture and pushed upwards, invaginating the detached fascia before it, and it must be made to enter the inguinal canal far enough to define the lower border of the internal oblique muscle stretched over it. A large curved needle (unarmed) is then passed on the finger as a guide, through the internal oblique tendon, the internal portion of the ring, and the skin of the abdomen; it is then threaded and withdrawn. Again, the needle (now with a thread) is guided by the finger and pushed through Poupart's ligament and the external pillar of the ring as before; while by a little manipulation its point is made to protrude through the same opening in the skin as before, a loop of thread is now left there, and the needle, still threaded, is again withdrawn. The next stitch, still guided on the finger, takes up the tendinous layer of the triangular aponeurosis covering the outer border of the rectus tendon close to the pubic spine; the point of the needle is then turned obliquely, so as to protrude through the original puncture in the skin a third time, the needle is then freed from the thread and withdrawn, thus leaving two ends and one intermediate loop of thread all at the one opening. These are so arranged that when they are tightened they draw together the sides of the canal; they are then secured over a compress of lint. The compress is removed and the stitches loosened, at dates varying from the third to the seventh day.

Mr. Wood now uses wire instead of thread. It has the advantage of greater firmness, excites less suppuration, and may be left much longer in situ, in consequence of which there is less risk of suppuration or pyæmia, and more chance of a good consolidation of the parts.

In congenital herniæ, and small ruptures in children and young boys, Mr. Wood uses rectangular pins in the following manner:—The scrotum being invaginated (without any incision through the skin) as far as possible up the canal, a rectangular pin, with a slightly-curved spear-pointed head, is passed through the skin of the groin to the operator's forefinger; guided by it, it is brought safely down the canal, and brought out through the skin of the scrotum just over the fundus of the hernial sac. A second pin is passed from the lower opening (still guided by the finger) in an upward direction, transfixing in its course the posterior surface of the outer pillar of the superficial ring, its point being brought out through, or at least close to, the first puncture made by the first pin. The pins are then locked in each other's loops— the punctures and skin protected by lint or adhesive plaster,— and the whole is retained by lint and a spica bandage. The pins should generally be withdrawn about the tenth day.

The author has now in many cases stitched with catgut the edges of the ring after the ordinary operation for hernia with the best effect.

2. *For Femoral Rupture.*—Cases suitable for operation are very infrequent; but should such a one be met with, Mr. Wood proposes the following operation on the same plan as the preceding. The hernia being fully reduced and the parts relaxed by position, an incision about an inch long should be made over the fundus of the tumour, and its edges raised so as to admit the finger fairly into the crural opening. The vein is then to be pushed inwards, and the needle passed through the pubic portion of the fascia lata of the thigh, and then through Poupart's ligament, appearing on the skin of the abdomen, a wire is then passed through the eye of the needle and hooked down, appearing through the wound, it is then withdrawn, and the needle again passed through the pubic portion of the fascia lata, but about three-quarters of an inch to the inside of the first puncture, then through Poupart's ligament again, and protruded through the same orifice in the skin; the other end of the wire is then hooked down as before, leaving a loop above, at the needle orifice, and two ends at the wound in the skin below. Both loops and ends must be managed as before.

> The author after operating for the relief of strangulation in a case of very large femoral hernia in a girl aged 23, stitched up the neck of the sac, and also stitched it to Gimbernat's ligament. The result for some months was admirable, though the hernia had been a very difficult one to replace from its size, and had been long in the habit of coming down. Eventually protrusion occurred to a very slight extent, but a truss keeps it completely up.

3. *For Umbilical Rupture.*—The principle involved in Mr. Wood's operation for umbilical rupture is precisely the same as for inguinal and crural. It consists in stitching the two edges of the tendinous aperture by wire; the needle is passed on a sort of small scoop or broad grooved director, which at once invaginates the skin and protects the bowel. Two stitches are thus inserted on each side. For the ingenious method by which they are introduced subcutaneously, I must refer to the detailed description in Mr. Wood's monograph. The wires are thus twisted and tightened over a pad of lint or wood, drawing together the edges of the opening in the tendon.

OPERATIONS FOR ARTIFICIAL ANUS.—In children the condition known as imperforate anus may sometimes be remedied by exploratory operations in the perineum, guided by the protrusion caused by the distended intestine. There are other cases, however, in which the rectum, as well as the anus, seems to be deficient, and in which, from the want of protrusion, there is no warrant for attempting an operation there; in these the only chance of life that remains is in an attempt to open the bowel higher up.

In adults, again, absolute closure of the rectum and anus, and complete obstruction, may be the result of malignant disease, or even, very rarely, of simple organic stricture.

175

In such cases, where the patient is tolerably strong and yet evidently doomed from the complete obstruction, an attempt at the formation of an artificial anus is warrantable, and in many cases afford great relief, and prolongs life for months.

Without going into all the various positions proposed for such operations, I select the two most warrantable, which have borne the test of experience. These are—1. Colotomy in the left loin. This is applicable in the case of adults with rectal obstruction. 2. Colotomy in the left groin applicable in cases of imperforate anus and deficiency of rectum in infants.

1. *Colotomy in the left loin*, generally known by the name of Amussat's operation.—The patient is laid upon his face, a pillow placed under the abdomen, rendering the left flank prominent. A transverse incision should then be made at a level about two finger-breadths above the crest of the ilium, extending from the outer edge of the erector spinæ muscle forward for four or five inches, according to the fatness of the patient; the muscles must then be carefully divided till the transversalis fascia is exposed. It is then to be pinched up and divided, as in the operation for strangulated hernia. The muscular wall of the colon uncovered by peritoneum is then in most cases very easily recognised from its immense distension. The bowel should then be hooked up by a curved needle, two or three points at least secured to the margins of the wounds by stitches, and then the bowel should be opened by a longitudinal incision of at least an inch in length. When the distension has been great, there is generally a rush of fluid fæces, which must be provided for, special care being taken lest any get into the cavity of the peritoneum.

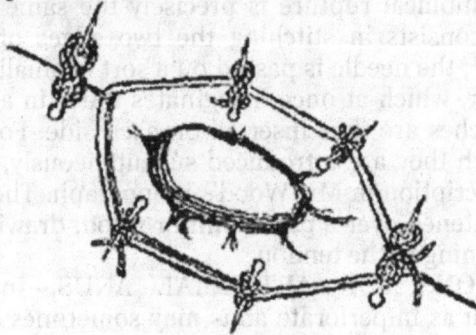

Fig. xxxiii.[147]

2. *Colotomy in the left groin*, for absence of anus and deficiency of rectum in newly born infants.—The dissections of Curling, Gosselin, and others have shown that in infants the operation of lumbar colotomy is very difficult, and its results uncertain, while it is

---

[147] Diagram of an artificial anus, showing small sutures which unite the edges of the gut and the skin, and the large ones stitching up the wound beyond.

176

comparatively easy to open the colon in the left groin. Huguier, again, has shown that in certain cases the colon is not to be found in the left groin, but is accessible in the right groin. This abnormality seems, as shown by Curling, to occur not oftener than once in every ten cases.

Operation.—An oblique incision from an inch and a half to two inches in length should be made in the left iliac region above Poupart's ligament, extending a little above the anterior-superior spinous process of the ilium. The fibres of the abdominal muscles should be divided on a director passed beneath them, and the peritoneum should next be cautiously opened to a sufficient extent. The colon will most likely protrude, but if small intestine appear the colon must be sought for higher up. A curved needle armed with a silk ligature should be passed lengthways through the coats of the upper part of the colon, and another inserted in the same way below, and the bowel, being drawn forwards, should then be opened by a longitudinal incision. The colon must afterwards be attached to the skin forming the margin of the wound by four sutures at the points of entry and exit of the needles.

OPERATION FOR THE REMOVAL OF AN ARTIFICIAL ANUS, in cases where the bowel is patent below.—After the operation for hernia in a case where the bowel is gangrenous, the only hope of the patient's recovery consists in the formation of adhesions between the bowel and the external wound, and the presence, for a time at least, of an artificial anus. If adhesions do form, and the patient recovers, it becomes a matter of great importance for his future comfort that the canal of the intestine should be re-established, and the fistulous opening allowed to close. This, however, is by no means easy, as even when the portion of intestine destroyed has been very small, a septum or valve remains which directs the contents of the bowel outwards, and so long as it exists is an effectual obstacle to any of the fæcal contents passing into the distal portion of the bowel. This septum or éperon is formed by the mesenteric side of the two ends of the bowel. To destroy this without causing peritonitis is the aim of the surgeon, and it is not an easy matter to accomplish. To cut it away would at once open the peritoneal cavity, so the mode of treatment now adopted in the rare cases where it is necessary is that recommended by Dupuytren. The principle of it is to destroy the éperon by pressure so gradual as to cause adhesive inflammation between the two surfaces, and thus seal up the cavity of the peritoneum, before the continuance of the same pressure shall have caused sloughing of the septum. This is managed by the gradual approximation by a screw of the blades of a pair of forceps, to which Dupuytren gave the name Enterotome. The process, which extends over days and weeks, must be carefully watched lest the inflammation go too far.

Plastic operations are occasionally required to close the opening after the passage is restored. For a good example of such an operation see Edin. Med. Journal for August 1873, in which Mr. John Duncan describes a case.

CHAPTER XII

OPERATIONS ON PELVIS

LITHOTOMY.—However interesting and even instructive it might be, any history of the various operations for the removal of calculi from the bladder would be quite out of place in a manual such as this. It will be sufficient here to describe the operations recommended and practised in the present day.

There are three different situations in which the bladder may be entered for the purpose of removing a calculus:—

1. The perineum, where access is gained through the urethra, prostate, and neck of the bladder.

2. Above the pubes, where the portion of bladder not covered by peritoneum is opened from above.

3. From the rectum.

1. LITHOTOMY THROUGH THE PERINEUM, by far the most frequent position for the operation.—Very various methods for its performance have been devised, differing in the nature and shape of the instruments employed, the direction and size of the incisions, the nature of the wound; but all resemble each other in certain very cardinal and important particulars. Thus all agree that it is absolutely necessary to enter the bladder at one spot—the neck of the bladder; and that to do this safely the urethra must be opened, and some instrument previously introduced by the urethra is to be used as a guide for the knife. But an instrument in the urethra and bladder is surrounded for at least an inch of its course by the prostate; and thus the knife, gorget, or finger, which, guided by the instrument in the urethra, is intended to cut or dilate the entrance to the bladder for the purpose of allowing the calculus to be removed, cannot do this without also cutting or dilating this prostate gland. Experience has proved that much of the success of the operation depends upon the position and amount of incision made in this prostate gland. But it might be asked, Why can we not enter the bladder by one side, avoiding altogether its neck and this prostate gland? For this, among other reasons, that the bladder normally contains, and so long as the patient lives must contain, a certain quantity of a very irritating fluid. It is surrounded by the loose areolar tissue of the pelvis, into which, if any of this fluid escapes, abcesses will form and death probably ensue; this result will almost certainly follow any opening made into the bladder except at one spot. This spot is the neck of the bladder. Why does urinary infiltration not occur there? Because the fascia of the pelvis (which when entire can resist infiltration) is prolonged forwards at the neck of the bladder, over the

prostate (Fig. xxxiv. pf), for which it forms a very strong funnel-like sheath. So long as this sheath is not cut where it covers the sides of the prostate, urinary infiltration of the pelvis is impossible, the urine being carried forwards and fairly out of the pelvis in this urine-tight funnel.

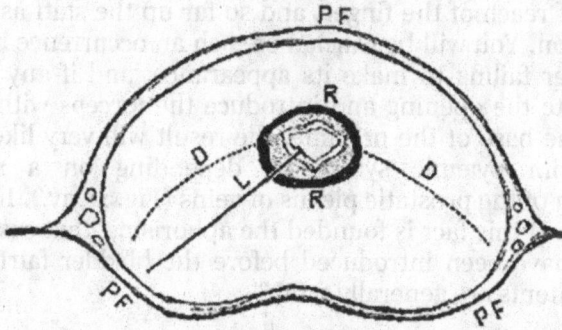

Fig.xxxiv.[148]

But it may now be said, If this be the case, we are very much limited in the size of the incision we may make into the bladder. We cannot remove a large stone, for the prostate ought not to be larger than a good-sized chestnut, and any cut we might make through a chestnut without cutting out of its side must be very small. Very true; but fortunately the sheath of the prostate, unlike the rind of the chestnut, is very freely dilatable, and will allow the passage of a very considerable stone.

Again, an inquirer might ask, If it is so dilatable, why should we run the risk of cutting the prostate at all? Why should we not introduce instruments gradually increasing in size into the membranous portion of the urethra, and thus dilate prostate and neck of bladder? For this reason, that the urethral canal passing through the prostate is itself lined immediately outside of the mucous membrane by a firm membranous sheath (Fig. xxxiv. rr), which resists dilatation to the utmost. Experience tells us that any attempts to dilate or even forcibly to tear this ring of fibrous texture are both ineffectual and dangerous, while a clean cut into it and through it into the substance of the prostate is at once effectual and comparatively safe.

In a word, we can describe the relation of the prostate to the operation of lithotomy somewhat in this manner:—Its fibrous sheath surrounding the urethra must be cut freely. The gland substance may be cut and freely dilated by the finger. Its fibrous envelope must, as far as possible, be preserved intact, but this interferes the less with the operation, as it is comparatively freely dilatable.

---

[148] Diagram of section of prostate seen from the inside:—pf, pelvic fascia or prostatic sheath; rr, ring which must be cut; l, position of incision in the lateral operation; dd, position of incisions in the bilateral operation.

179

The firm lining of the urethra, which must be cut, is specially strong at its base, forming a tough resisting band just at the aperture of the bladder, which, unfortunately, is often so high up in the pelvis in tall patients, or in cases in which the prostate is much enlarged, as to be almost out of reach of the finger, and so far up the staff as perhaps to escape division. You will be warned of such an occurrence by the urine in the bladder failing to make its appearance; and if any attempt be made to dilate the opening and introduce the forceps without further incision of the base of the prostate, the result will very likely be fatal, generally from pyæmic symptoms depending on a suppurative inflammation of the prostatic plexus of veins (Fig. xxxiv.). In fact, upon a recognition of this fact is founded the aphorism, "that cases in which the forceps have been introduced before the bladder fairly begins to empty its contents are generally fatal."

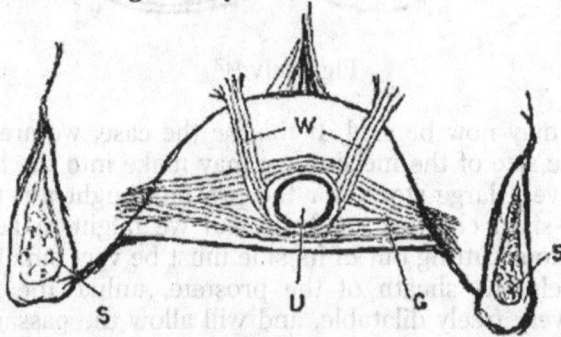

Fig. xxxv.[149]

We have thus traced the necessary guiding principles as to our incisions from the bladder outwards through the prostatic portion of the urethra. We have next to discover what sort of an opening is necessary in the membranous portion of the urethra consistent with the fulfilment of the same conditions, namely, freedom of escape for the urine, and room enough to remove the stone. Both of these are gained at once by a free incision of the membranous portion, dividing especially those anterior fibres of the great sphincter muscle of the pelvis, the levator ani, which embrace the membranous portion, under the special names of compressor (Fig. xxv.) and levator urethræ (Guthrie's and Wilson's muscles).

The principles which guide the position and size of the preliminary incisions which enable the urethra to be opened are very simple:—(1.) The wound in the perineum should be large enough to give free access to the urethra, and easy egress to the stone; (2.) It

[149] Diagram of muscles of membranous portion of urethra seen from the inside:— ss, section of os pubis; u, urethra; g, Guthrie's muscle, compressor urethræ; w, Wilson's muscle, levator urethræ.

should be conical, with its base outwards, so as to favour escape of urine and prevent infiltration; (3.) It should not wound any important organ or vessel; that is, it must avoid the rectum, the corpus spongiosum, especially the bulb, if possible, the artery of the bulb, and in every case should leave the pudic artery intact.

So far for broad general principles, which must guide all methods of successful lithotomy.

THE LATERAL OPERATION.—*Operation of Cheselden.*—(1.) *Instruments required.*—A staff with a broad substantial handle, and a longer curve than the ordinary catheter requires, furnished with a very deep and wide groove, which occupies the space midway between its convexity and its left side. The one used should invariably be large enough to dilate fully the urethra.

A knife, with its blade three or four inches in length, but sharp only for an inch and a half from its point, its back straight up to within a sixth of an inch of its point, and there deflected at an angle to the point, which again curves to the edge. The angle from the back to the point permits the knife to run more freely along the groove in the staff.

A probe-pointed straight knife with a narrow blade may occasionally be useful in enlarging the incision in the prostate, when this is required by the size of the stone.

Forceps of various sizes and shapes, some with the blades curved at an angle to reach stones lying behind an enlarged prostate, all with broad blades as thin as is consistent with perfect inflexibility, the blades hollowed and roughened in the inside, but without the projecting teeth sometimes recommended, which are dangerous from being apt to break the stone.

A scoop to remove fragments or small stones, sometimes useful with the aid of the forefinger in lifting out a large one.

A flexible tube of at least half an inch calibre, and about six inches long, rounded off and fenestrated above, fitted at its outer end with a ring and two eyelet-holes for the tapes, with which it is tied into the bladder.

Prior to the operation the patient's health should be attended to, the stomach and bowels regulated, and any disorder of the kidneys or bladder as far as possible alleviated. If his health has been good and habits active, three or four days' confinement to his room on low diet, with a full purge the evening before the operation, is all the preparatory treatment that is necessary.

It is of the utmost importance for the safety of the operation and the patient's comfort after it, that the rectum be completely unloaded before the operation, and the bowels so far emptied as to permit three or four days after the operation to elapse without any movement of the bowels being necessary. If there is any doubt as to the effect of the laxative, a large stimulant enema should be administered on the morning of the operation.

181

Position.—Much depends on the proper tying up of the patient. He should be placed with his breech projecting over the edge of a narrow table, with head slightly raised on a pillow, but the shoulders low. The hands are then to be secured each to its corresponding foot, by a strong bandage passing round wrist and instep, or by suitable leather anklets, the knees should be wide apart, and on exactly the same level, so that the pelvis may be quite straight. An assistant should be placed to take charge of each leg.

The staff is next introduced and the stone felt; if there is little water in the bladder a few ounces may be injected, but this is rarely necessary, for the patient should be ordered to retain as much water as possible, and when he cannot retain it, injection of water may do harm, and will probably not be retained, but at once come away along the groove in the staff. The staff is then committed to a special assistant, who must be thoroughly up to his duty, and attend to the staff alone.

Some surgeons direct the assistant to make the convexity of the staff bulge in the perineum, to enable the groove to be struck more easily. It will be, however, safer both for the rectum and the bulb, if the staff be hooked firmly up against the symphysis pubis, as advised by Liston. The same assistant can also keep the scrotum up out of the way.

If the perineum has not been previously shaved, this is now done.

The operator sits down on a low stool in front of the patient's breech, his instruments being ready to his hand, and then steadying the skin of the perineum with the fingers of his left hand, enters the point of the knife in the raphe of the perineum, midway between the anus and scrotum (one inch in front of anus—Cheselden, Crichton; one and a quarter—Gross, Skey, and Brodie; one and three-quarters—Fergusson; one inch behind the scrotum—Liston), and carries the incision obliquely downwards and outwards, in a line midway between the anus and tuberosity of the ischium. The length of the incision must vary with the size of the perineum, and the supposed size of the stone, but there is less risk in its being too large, so long as the rectum is safe, than in its being too small. Its depth should be greatest at its upper angle, where it has to divide the parts to the depth of the transverse muscle of the perineum, and least at its lower angle, where a deep incision is not required, and would be almost sure to wound the rectum.

The forefinger of the left hand is now to be deeply inserted into the wound, and any remaining fibres of the levator ani in front are to be divided, the edge of the knife being directed from above downwards. The left forefinger being still used to push its way through the cellular tissue, the groove in the staff is now felt in the membranous portion of the urethra covered by the deep fascia of the perineum. Now comes the deeper part of the incision. Guided by the finger-nail of the left hand, the surgeon introduces the point of the knife into the groove of the staff. He then takes hold of the staff for a moment to feel that it is held up properly against the pubis, and in the middle line, and also that the knife is fairly in the groove. Giving the staff back again to the assistant, and keeping the rectum well out of the way by the left hand, he now steadily directs the knife along the groove of the staff till the bladder is fairly entered, and the ring at the base of the prostate completely divided. When this is the case a gush of urine takes place, following the withdrawal of the knife.

When making the deep incision, and in the groove of the staff, the blade of the knife should lie neither vertical nor horizontal, but midway between the two, so as to make the section of the left lobe of the prostate in its longest diameter, that is, in a direction downwards and backwards (Fig. xxxiv. L).

The knife is now withdrawn, and the left forefinger inserted. In most cases it will be long enough to reach the bladder and touch the stone, and may then be freely used by gradual pressure to dilate the wound; this may be done very freely when necessary for a large stone, if only the ring of fibrous tissue surrounding the urethra be first cut and the bladder fairly entered. Whenever the stone is felt by the finger, the assistant may withdraw the staff.

When the operator has thus felt the stone and sufficiently dilated the wound, the next step is to introduce the forceps; this should be done under the guidance of the finger, and with the blades closed. When the stone is felt the blades should be opened very widely, slightly withdrawn, and then pushed in again, the lower one, if possible, being insinuated under the stone. The blades must be made fairly to grasp and contain the stone in their hollow, for if they only nibble at the end of an oval stone, extraction is impossible. Extraction should then be performed slowly, with alternate wrigglings of the forceps from side to side, so as gradually to dilate, not to tear, the prostate, and the operator must remember to pull in the axis of the pelvis, not against the os pubis or the promontory of the sacrum.

If there is much resistance, it may possibly be caused by the stone having been caught in its longer axis, and this may be remedied by careful manipulation by means of the finger and forceps. If the stone is still too large to be extracted without greater force than is warrantable, there are still various expedients (see infra, pp. 265, 270).

In most cases, however, the stone is removed rapidly enough by the single incision. The finger, or a sound, must then be introduced to feel if any more stones are present. The closed forceps make a very effectual instrument for this purpose. Much information may be gained from the appearance of the first stone, the presence or absence of facets. Its smoothness or roughness enables us to form a pretty certain opinion; yet the bladder should always be carefully searched; and if the stone has been friable or broken in extraction, should be washed out by a current of water. Where the calculi are very numerous, or where many fragments have separated, the scoop will be found useful, both for detecting and removing them. All the stones being extracted, there is in most cases little or no bleeding (see infra, Hæmorrhage). The tube already described may now be inserted and tied into the bladder. It may be retained for forty-eight or seventy-two hours, according to circumstances. Care must be taken lest it be closed up by coagula during the first hour or two after the operation. In children the tube is not necessary, and from their restlessness might possibly do harm, but in adults (though neglected by some surgeons) experience shows it is a valuable adjunct in the after-treatment.

Having thus traced the course of an ordinary uncomplicated case of lithotomy by the lateral operation, a brief notice is suitable of some of the obstacles and difficulties, some of the dangers and bad results which may be met with, and the best methods of overcoming them.

1. *Large size of the stone*, as an obstacle to extraction. When, either from the enormous size of the stone, generally to be made out before the operation, or from some congenital or acquired deformity of the pelvis, it is obvious beforehand that the calculus cannot pass through the bony pelvis entire, a choice of two courses remains, either—

(1.) The high or supra-pubic operation (q.v. infra); or (2.) Crushing of the calculus in the bladder, and removal piecemeal. Instruments of great strength have been devised for this latter operation. The risk to the bladder is very great, and fragments are apt to be left behind; these are sure to form nuclei of new calculi.

2. *Peculiarities in the position or relations of the stone* in the bladder:—

(1.) It may lie in a sort of pouch behind the prostate, and thus be out of the reach of the forceps. This may be remedied by the use of curved forceps, or, better still, by the finger in the rectum to tilt up the stone into the bladder.

(2.) It may lie above the pubis in the anterior wall of the bladder. Pressure on the hypogastrium, or the use of a strong probe as a hook, will generally suffice to dislodge it.

(3.) The stone may be encysted. This is extremely rare, and, as Fergusson says, we hear more of these from bunglers who have operated only several times, than from those who have had large experience.

3. *An enlarged prostate* is at once a source of difficulty and of some danger.

The distance of the bladder from the surface may be so very much increased by enlargement of the prostate as to render even the longest forefinger too short to reach the stone or even the bladder. This renders the introduction of the forceps more difficult and uncertain, the dilatation more prolonged, and the extraction more dangerous. If very large, the groove of the staff may not reach the bladder, and thus the deep incision may fail of cutting the ring at the base of the gland,

and the urine may thus not escape, and all the dangers of laceration of the ring may result. Such cases may be well managed by the insertion of a straight deeply grooved staff into the insufficient incision, and fairly into the bladder, and on this, pushing a cutting gorget through the uncut portion of the gland. This insures a sufficient yet not dangerous incision, which we cannot so safely perform with the knife, as the parts are so far beyond the reach of the guiding forefinger.

Under the head of risks after lithotomy we may class the following:—

1. Sinking, or shock. In the very aged or very young, or after a very prolonged or painful operation, shock may now and then kill the patient within a few hours. Since the days of chloroform this result is extremely rare.

2. Hæmorrhage seems to be a very infrequent risk. The transverse perineal artery, which is always cut in the operation, is small, and rarely bleeds much. If the bulb is wounded, as no doubt frequently occurs, the flow from it can easily be checked. The pudic is so well protected from any ordinary incision as to be practically safe; and if wounded by some frightfully extensive incision, it can be compressed against the tuberosity of the ischium.

There is an abnormal distribution of the dorsal artery of the penis, in which, rising higher up than it ought, and coursing along the neck of the bladder, and the lateral lobe of the prostate, it may be divided. This may give trouble, and even result in fatal hæmorrhage. Fortunately it is rare. The author has met with one case in a boy of eleven, in whom a very severe hæmorrhage was not to be explained. The patient recovered without another bad symptom.

Again, a general oozing may often appear a few hours after the operation, when the patient is warm in bed, apparently from the substance of the prostate. If raising the breech and the application of cold fail to arrest it, it may be necessary to plug the wound. This is done by stuffing it with long strips of lint round the tube. Great care must be then taken lest the tube become occluded.

3. Infiltration of urine may occur as a result of a too free incision of the vesical fascia (in adults), and still more frequently of a too small external wound.

Here it should be noticed that in children it is fortunately of very little consequence to preserve the integrity of the prostatic sheath of vesical fascia. In them the prostate is so exceedingly small and undeveloped, that even the forefinger could not be introduced into the bladder without a complete section of the prostate. Probably from the blander nature of their urine, and the greater vitality of their tissues, this is of less consequence, as it is rarely found that any bad effects result from this section.

Among other risks we find peritonitis, inflammation of neck of bladder, inflammation of prostatic plexus of veins, resulting in pyæmia, suppression of urine, and other kidney complications. For the symptoms and treatment of these there is no place in a mere manual of surgical operations.

Wound of rectum and recto-vesical fistula.—Such wounds were not uncommon, and in many cases unavoidable, before the days of chloroform, from the struggles of the patient; now they are comparatively rare, and should be still rarer. They probably occur in more cases than the surgeon is aware of, and heal up without his knowledge; we may arrive at this conclusion from the fact that small wounds are found in post-mortem examinations of cases in which no such complication has been thought of.

They occasionally heal without giving any trouble, but, at other times, as the external wound contracts, a communication forms between rectum and the urethra, in which the contents are apt to be interchanged in a most disagreeable manner, flatus passing per urethram, and urine per rectum.

When it is evidently not going to heal spontaneously, the septum between the external orifice of the wound and the communication with the gut should be laid open, as in the operation for fistula in ano.

There are certain modifications and varieties in the method of operating for stone through the perineum, which deserve at least a brief notice:—

1. *The bilateral operation.*—Though he was not the inventor, Dupuytren's name is justly associated with this operation. The principle of it is to divide both sides of the prostate equally, so as to give more room for extraction of a large stone, without the necessity of much laceration, or the risk of cutting through the prostatic sheath of fascia.

The operation.—A semilunar incision is made transversely across the perineum, extending from a point midway between the right tuber ischii and the anus, upwards, crossing the raphe nearly an inch above the anus, and then curving downwards to a corresponding point on the opposite side. The skin, superficial fascia, and a few of the anterior fibres of the external sphincter, are thus divided, and the groove of the staff sought by the forefinger. The membranous portion of the urethra is then laid open in the middle line, and the beak of a double lithotome caché securely lodged in the groove. It is then pushed into the bladder with its concavity upwards, and when fairly in it is turned round, its blades protruded to the required extent, and withdrawn with its concavity downwards, thus dividing both lobes of the prostate in a direction downwards and outwards (Fig. xxiv. D D). The operation is finished in the usual manner. Though it is a comparatively easy operation, and theoretically may be proved to have many advantages, experience has shown that the results are not so favourable as those of the ordinary lateral operation.

2. Buchanan's medio-lateral operation on a rectangular staff.—The staff is bent at a right angle three inches from the end, and deeply grooved on its left side. This is introduced into the urethra so that the angle projects the membranous portion of the urethra close to the apex of the prostate and the terminal straight portion enters the bladder parallel to the rectum. The angle projects in the perineum, so that the operator with his left forefinger in the rectum is enabled, by a stab with a long straight bistoury (held horizontally and with the cutting edge to the left side), at once to enter the groove, and, by following the groove, the bladder. Whenever the escape of urine shows that the bladder is fairly reached, the knife is withdrawn so as to make a lateral section of the prostate, and then, with the finger still in the rectum, to make an incision in the ischio-rectal fossa, of sufficient size to allow the stone to be easily withdrawn.

The inventor claims for this method that it is easier, that there is less risk of hæmorrhage, wound of the rectum, and infiltration of urine.

3. *Allarton's operation of median lithotomy* suits admirably for stones known to be small, but is quite unsuitable for large ones. Probably in most cases it should be superseded by lithotrity.

Operation.—A large curved staff with a central groove is to be held firmly hooked up against the symphysis pubis, and then steadied by the left forefinger in the rectum. The operator pierces the raphe of the perineum with a long straight bistoury about half an inch above the verge of the anus, enters the groove of the staff, and cuts inwards, almost, but not quite, into the bladder. In withdrawing the knife the wound in the urethra is enlarged upwards towards the scrotum. A ball-pointed probe is then passed on the staff into the bladder, the staff is withdrawn, and the finger, guided by the probe, is used to dilate the neck of the bladder, to an extent sufficient for the removal of the stone by a small pair of forceps.

In this operation the prostate is hardly incised at all. The results are not better than those of the lateral operation.

2. LITHOTOMY ABOVE THE PUBES, *or the High Operation.*— In cases where, from the known size of the stone, or from the deformity of the bones of the pelvis, it is impossible that the stone can be extracted entire in the usual manner; in cases where the prostate is very much enlarged, or where there is any real or supposed likelihood of inflammation of the neck of the bladder, the supra-pubic operation may be warrantable. Its performance is easy, it does not involve any wound of the peritoneum if properly performed, and there is no risk of hæmorrhage. There are certainly great risks attending it of peritonitis and urinary infiltration.

In more than one case this operation has been attended by

wound of peritoneum and subsequent escape of intestines through the wound, even when dressed antiseptically and performed under spray.

Operation.—The patient lies on his back, with his head and shoulders slightly raised, so as to relax the abdominal muscles, and his legs hanging down over the edge of the table. If his bladder can bear it, it should be fully distended, either by voluntary retention of the urine, or by injection with tepid water. A vertical incision is then made in the middle line, separating the recti muscles from below upwards, care being taken to push the peritoneum well out of the way, which is easily done by the finger in the loose cellular tissue of the part. The anterior wall of the bladder is then exposed, uncovered by peritoneum; it must be opened with great care, also in the middle line, while the wound in the parietes is held aside by retractors. The wall of the bladder should be transfixed by a curved needle, and thus held in position before it is opened. The stone is then removed by a pair of straight forceps, generally with great ease. Attempts used to be made to leave a catheter or canula in the bladder wound to prevent infiltration. Probably the safest method now will be to close the bladder wound at once by metallic stitches, and stitching the abdominal wound carefully with deeply entered wires, to leave the patient on his back. When compared with the lateral operations the statistics of the supra-pubic operation are discouraging, the mortality being one in three and a half to one in four. But in cases where the stone is known to be very large and of firm consistence, the risks are probably less from this method than from lateral lithotomy, followed by efforts to crush the stone through the wound prior to its removal.

The late Mr. George Bell, a most successful lithotomist, proposed to perform this operation in two stages. In a case of greatly enlarged prostate, where the bladder had been punctured above the pubes by a country surgeon for retention of urine, he dilated the track of the canula by means of sponge-tents gradually increased in size, and then succeeded in extracting through the dilated opening several large calculi. The case recovered, and may encourage similar attempts.

3. OPERATIONS THROUGH THE RECTUM.—(a.) Sanson's Recto-vesical Operation.—The principle of this operation consisted in laying the two canals, the rectum and the urethra, into one. A large staff, grooved on its convexity, being inserted into the urethra, the operator, with the forefinger of his left hand in the rectum as a guide to the knife, pierces the anterior wall of the rectum, reaches the groove of the staff just in front of the prostate, and cutting outwards divides the rectum, the anterior fibres of levator ani, and the sphincter, as well as the skin of the perineum in the middle line. Entering the knife again into the groove of the staff, it is to be pushed right onwards into the bladder, dividing the prostate, and avoiding if possible the seminal vesicles and ducts; the stone is then very easily removed.

Though this operation was supposed to lessen the risk of pelvic infiltration it is not found to do so, and it adds the additional inconvenience of almost inevitable rectal fistula, through which the urine escapes. It is certainly a very easy operation, but the mortality is found to be greater than in the ordinary lateral operation.

(b.) *Lithotomy through the rectum above the prostate.*—The presence of a small portion of bladder beyond the prostate in close relation to the rectum renders it possible, in cases where the prostate is not enlarged, to enter the bladder and remove a stone of moderate size, without interfering with the peritoneum, prostate, or neck of the bladder.

This ingenious but difficult operation was performed for the first time by Drs. Sims and Bauer in 1859.

I quote the brief notice of the operation by Dr. Sims from the Lancet of 1864 (vol. i. p. 111):—

"The patient was placed on the left side, and my speculum was introduced into the rectum, exposing the anterior wall of the rectum, just as it would the vagina in the female. A sound was passed into the bladder. The doctor entered the blade of a bistoury in the triangular space bounded by the prostate, the vesiculæ seminales, and the peritoneal reduplication. He passed the finger through this opening, felt the stone, and removed it with the forceps without the least trouble. The operation was done as quickly and as easily as it would have been in a female through the vaginal septum. After the removal of the stone, Dr. Bauer kindly asked me to close the wound with silver sutures, which I did, introducing some five or six wires, with the same facility as in the vagina. There was no leakage of urine. The patient recovered without the least trouble of any sort. The wires were removed on the eighth day, and on the ninth day the patient rode in a carriage with Dr. Bauer a distance of four or five miles, to call on, and report himself to, our distinguished countryman, Dr. Mott."

The chief risks in this operation seem to be the chance of wounding the peritoneal cul-de-sac, as the amount of free space between it and the prostate seems to vary much in individuals and in races. Dr. Marion Sims mentioned to me in conversation that he believed this operation impossible in the negro race, from the greater projection downwards of the peritoneal reduplication. An enlarged prostate would be an insuperable objection. The use of silver wire, to close up the wound at once, diminishes very much any risk of recto-vesical fistula.

LITHOTRITY OR LITHOTRIPSY.—There exist cases of stone in the bladder, which, under certain conditions, may be relieved without lithotomy, by an operation which crushes the stone into fragments small enough to be discharged through the urethra.

To enter with any fulness into the history, literature, and varieties of this operation, and the instruments required, would in itself require a large volume. Suffice it here to describe the case suitable for the operation, the essentials required in the instrument, and the method of performance.

1. *For a case to be suitable* the stone should not be too large, and especially not too hard, also there should not be too many of them.

The urethra should be capacious enough to let the instrument pass easily and painlessly.

The bladder should be large enough to contain four ounces of water at least, should not be much inflamed, and, on the other hand, should not be paralysed. Paralysis or want of tone in the bladder prevents the thorough evacuation of its contents, and still more the expulsion of the fragments of stone.

2. *A good instrument* should, as far as possible, combine strength with lightness. The curved portion of the fixed blade should be fenestrated to allow escape of the fragments and thorough closure of the instrument.

The movable blade must be so arranged as to combine perfect ease of movement up and down in seeking for the stone, with a powerful, slow, and gradual approximation in crushing it. This can be managed by an ingenious arrangement, which leaves the movable blade under the control only of the operator's thumb till the stone is found, and yet, by touching a spring, gives him the advantage either of a fine screw or of a rack and pinion movement for crushing the stone.

3. *Operation.*—The patient being prepared by a free evacuation of the bowels, and the urethra having been previously fairly dilated, he is asked to retain his urine as long as possible, or, if he cannot do so, a few ounces of tepid water may be injected per urethram.

He is then laid on a sofa or table, the breech being well raised by pillows, the shoulders low, the thighs and knees bent up and separated. The instrument, well warmed and oiled, is then introduced with the blades closed. When fairly into the bladder the search for the stone begins.

There are differences of opinion regarding the best method of fishing for the stone; great patience and gentleness, with a thorough previous acquaintance with bladder manipulation, are required, whichever method be chosen.

The two chief methods may be described as the English and the French, the latter, Civiale's, being now used by Sir Henry Thompson, and other English operators. Briefly, the two are:—

(1.) *Heurteloup's and Sir B. C. Brodie's.*—In this, after the instrument is fairly entered, its handle is elevated, thus depressing the curved extremity, the forceps are then opened, and, by being kept as low as possible in the bladder, it is hoped that the calculus will fall into the opened blades by its own weight. In this method the fundus is the scene of crushing, and there is a risk of injuring the sensitive neck of the bladder, especially at the moment of opening the blades.

(2.) *Civiale's—Thompson's.*—In this the pelvis is to be so elevated that the centre of the bladder and space beneath it give plenty of room for seizing the stone, and all contact with the wall of the bladder is (as far as possible) avoided.

The instrument is introduced closed, and carried fairly away in to the posterior part of the bladder before it is opened at all. It probably grazes the stone in passing, and, if so, is directed to the side of the bladder in which the stone is not lying. Then when nearly touching the posterior wall, the movable blade is withdrawn, the instrument inclined towards the stone lying unmoved in the most dependent part, and there seizes it generally with ease.

If not felt, the blades are again to be opened, turned a little to the other side of the bladder, and then closed. Sir H. Thompson lays the greatest stress on the importance of always having the blades fairly opened before shifting their position, for if moved when closed, the very opening of the movable blade is certain to drive the stone out of the way and prevent its seizure.

Certain rules are useful:—Move the axis of the instrument as little as possible; it should be kept in the centre of the bladder, so far in, that the movements of the male blade are quite free from the neck of the bladder and prostate, and the blades only should be moved in the bladder on the centre of the shaft as an axis. There should be no jerking once the stone is caught, and the crushing should be done as far as possible in the very centre of the bladder, the blades not touching any of the walls.

After the stone is seized, do not crush till, by a turn of the blades from side to side, you discover that none of the mucous membrane of the bladder is caught in the instrument.

The lithotrite is not meant to extract stones, but to crush them, hence never attempt to withdraw it unless the blades are in absolute apposition.

Never attempt too much at one time. Sir H. Thompson holds that five minutes is the longest time that should be given, perhaps in most cases three minutes being long enough.

While many surgeons will still agree with the above advice, Dr. Bigelow of Boston has lately been highly commending a method which he has called Litholapaxy, in which, at one sitting under chloroform, the stone is crushed and aspirated, or sucked out of the bladder at once.[150]

Since the above was written the operation of Litholapaxy has made great strides in the favour of surgeons, and many stones that would have been removed by lithotomy are now broken down by powerful instruments at a single sitting, and removed piecemeal by the suction apparatus.

---

[150] Boston Medical and Surgical Journal, May 29, 1879.

S. W. Gross has collected 312 cases, of which 17 died or 5.45 per cent., but of 180 done by experienced surgeons, Thompson, Bigelow, Van Buren, Weir, and Stevenson only five died, or 3.33 per cent., while of 1470 cases of lithotrity, as formerly practised, 159, or 10.81, per cent. died.[151]

OPERATIONS FOR STRICTURE OF URETHRA.—Under this head many manipulations and operations might be described; the very instruments devised being exceedingly numerous and complicated. Enough here to detail a few of the more simple and practical procedures under the different heads of—1. Dilatation gradual and forced. 2. Internal Division. 3. External Division.

1. DILATATION.—Under this head we have—

a. *Vital dilatation.*—The passing of a succession of bougies, gradually increasing in diameter, at intervals of three or four days, for the purpose of exciting an amount of interstitial absorption in the new material constituting the stricture, sufficient to remove it. Passing a bougie, though certainly often very difficult, perhaps should hardly come into the category of surgical operations, yet to preserve a certain completeness in the account of stricture, a very brief description may be here inserted.

The recumbent posture is in most cases to be preferred. The patient should lie flat on his back, with the knees slightly bent and separated, and the head and shoulders slightly raised on a pillow. The operator standing on the patient's left side, raises the penis in his left hand, and with the right introduces the instrument, previously warmed and oiled, into the meatus. He then pushes it very gently onwards, at the same time stretching the penis with the left hand, just so far as to efface any wrinkles in the mucous membrane, till the point reaches the bulbous portion. The axis of the instrument, which at first for convenience was over the left groin, has now gradually been approaching the middle line. When this is reached, the instrument should be raised from the abdomen, and the handle cautiously carried in the arc of a circle first upwards and then downwards, till, when the instrument is fairly into the bladder, the handle is depressed between the patient's thighs. While this is being done the operator's left hand should be withdrawn from the penis, and the points of the fingers applied to the perineum.

In cases of difficulty certain points may be remembered:—

(1.) That the point of the instrument may in the first inch or two be occasionally entangled in a lacuna in the roof, especially when a small instrument is used; hence the beak should be at first maintained against the inferior wall of the canal.[152]

---

[151] Gross, Surgery, 6th ed. vol. ii. p. 736.
[152] Holmes's Surgery, vol. iv. p. 392.

(2.) That the handle should not be depressed too soon; if it is, there is a risk of a false passage being made through the upper wall.

(3.) The opposite error may force the point out of the urethra between the membranous portion and the rectum, and onwards into the substance of the prostate gland.

And certain cautions may be given:—

(1.) In every exploration of an unknown urethra the surgeon should commence with an instrument of medium size, certainly not less than No. 7 or 8.

(2.) In cases of difficulty occurring in the urethra behind the scrotum, invariably use the forefinger of the left hand in the rectum as a guide.

(3.) Expression of pain on the part of the patient is no indication that a false passage is being made, nor its absence that the instrument is in the passage, for it is a remark of Mr. Syme, that passing an instrument through a stricture is generally more painful than making a false passage through the walls of the urethra.

> An instrument may be passed, while the patient is erect, with the following precautions:—The patient should stand with his back against a wall, his arms supported on the back of a chair on each side, heels eight or ten inches apart, and four or five inches from the wall; his clothes thoroughly down, not merely opened. The bougie should then be held nearly horizontal, with its concavity over the left groin of the patient, the penis being raised in the surgeon's left hand. Introduced thus for four or five inches, the handle is gradually raised into the middle line of the abdomen, and to the perpendicular; it is then to be lightly depressed, and, as the point enters the bladder, brought down towards the operator until it sinks beneath the horizontal line.

b. *Mechanical dilatation* is of two kinds, both very rarely used:— (1.) When an instrument cannot be passed, it consists of passing down day after day the point of an instrument (sometimes armed with caustic, sometimes not), and pressing it against the stricture till it is overcome.[153] (2.) When an instrument is introduced through an intractable stricture, and is left there either for some hours, or for some days, to excite what is called "suppuration" of the stricture.[154]

c. Forced dilatation.—Under this head we might describe at great length mechanical contrivances to force or rupture a stricture. A word or two on a few of the most important:—

(1.) Conical bougies of steel or silver.

(2.) Mr. Wakley's method, on which many others have been founded. He passed a small bougie or wire into the bladder, over which

---

[153] See Miller's Practice of Surgery, p. 212.
[154] Solly's Surgical Experiences, pp. 537, 538, etc.

were slipped straight tubes of varying size, with perfect certainty that they could not leave the urethra.

(3.) Mr. Holt's method.[155]—The principle of it is to rupture the stricture at once, so that a No. 12 catheter can immediately be passed into the bladder.

He attains this object by means of an instrument composed of two grooved blades, united about one inch from their apex, into a conical sound, which at its apex is about the size of a No. 2 bougie. This is passed into the bladder, and the grooved blades are separated to any extent that is desired by passing down between them a straight rod equal in size of a No. 8, 10, or 12, bougie. To guide this properly it is made hollow, and it is passed down over a central wire which lies between the grooved blades of the instrument and is welded to the apex. A great improvement is effected on Mr. Holt's later instruments by this wire being made hollow, and fitted with a stilette, for by this means we can with certainty ascertain whether or not the instrument has been passed into the bladder. This instrument, which is an improvement upon one invented by Perrève nearly forty years ago, has been used on very many occasions by Mr. Holt and others with success. The risk to life, if the case be properly managed, is trifling, but, like every other means of treating stricture, it has the objection that the stricture is liable to recur, unless bougies be passed at intervals for months and years.

Sir Henry Thompson has introduced and described another very ingenious instrument for the same purpose, constructed on somewhat similar principles. His account of it, to which I must refer, will be found in Holmes's System of Surgery, 1st ed. vol. iv. p. 399.

2. INTERNAL DIVISION OF STRICTURE is a mode of treatment which by many surgeons is highly disapproved, yet of late years it has been more used than formerly, especially in resilient strictures. It may be done in two ways:—

(1.) *From before backwards.*—This method, to be at all admissible, requires a guide to be previously passed; a lancet-shaped blade may then be slipped down a groove in this guide till the stricture is divided. This is least objectionable in cases of stricture close to the meatus.

(2.) *From behind forwards.*—To make the incision thus, it is of course necessary that the stricture should be so far dilatable as to admit an instrument the point of which is large enough to contain the blade by which the stricture is to be divided. This will be found to be at least equal in size to a No. 3 or No. 4 catheter. In many instruments it is much larger.

Civiale's instrument for internal incision of the urethra from

---

[155] The Immediate Treatment of Stricture. By Bernard Holt, F.R.C.S. London. Third Edition, 1868.

behind forwards has the very high recommendation of Sir H. Thompson.[156] It consists of a sound with a bulbous extremity (as large as a No. 5 bougie) which contains a small blade, which can be made to project for such a distance as the operator wishes. It is passed through the stricture with the blade concealed, till the bulb is carried about one-third of an inch or more beyond the stricture; the blade is then projected, and the incision made by drawing it slowly but firmly outwards towards the meatus, with the blade towards the floor of the urethra, till the stricture is divided in its whole extent. Sir H. Thompson recommends this to be used in cases where it is not that the stricture is of very small calibre, but that it is undilatable, that prevents the cure. Many modifications of above have been devised by Lund, Teevan, and other surgeons, on similar principles.

3. MR. SYME'S OPERATION OF EXTERNAL DIVISION.—Mr. Syme held that no stricture through which the water can escape should be called impermeable, for by patience and care the surgeon should always be able to pass a slender director through the stricture on which it may be divided with ease and certainty. The old operation of "perineal section" for so-called impermeable stricture is very different, being difficult, dangerous, and uncertain in its results.

Operation.—A director is passed into the stricture. Mr. Syme's directors are of different sizes, the smallest being in diameter less than an ordinary surgical probe. They are made of steel, are grooved on the convexity, and have this peculiarity, that while the lower half is small, the upper is of full size (No. 8 or 10), the difference in calibre occurring quite abruptly. The presence of this "shoulder" on the staff enables the operator to ascertain exactly the position of the stricture, and also to tell when it is fully divided without the necessity of withdrawing the instrument.

This being fairly in the stricture, the patient is put in the position for lithotomy, an assistant holds the staff in his right hand, drawing up the scrotum with his left.

The surgeon then makes an incision in the middle line over the stricture for the necessary distance, from above downwards, till he exposes the urethra, and feels exactly the shoulder of the staff. Care must be taken not to go past the urethra at either side. When he distinctly feels the outline of the staff, he takes it in his left hand, and a short sharp-pointed bistoury in his right. It should be held firmly in the palm of the hand, with the back of the blade resting on the forefinger, the pulp of which guides the point to the groove, and guards it when making the incision; the knife is to be placed on the groove beyond (on the bladder side) of the stricture, and brought forwards, slowly cutting through the whole stricture; till the shoulder of the staff is reached. It

---

[156] Holmes's System of Surgery, 1st ed. vol. iv. p. 403.

195

requires strength and precision to divide thoroughly the indurated stricture, which is apt to elude the knife.

The shoulder of the staff can now be passed through the stricture if the operation is complete; if not, the incision must be extended, always in the middle line, and guided by the groove. When thoroughly divided, the staff is now to be withdrawn, and a full-sized catheter with a double curve passed into the bladder. This should not be furnished with a stop-cock or plug, lest the bladder should by inadvertence be allowed to be too full, and extravasation into the cellular tissue of the urethra take place along the side of the instrument.

The catheter should be tied in, and left for two, sometimes for three days, when it can generally be removed with safety, and a bougie should be passed at intervals of three or four, till the wound is healed. To prevent recurrence of the stricture, it is a wise precaution to pass an instrument at intervals for many months after the cure is apparently complete.

In certain cases, where the stricture is far back and the urinary symptoms severe, Mr. Syme found advantage from the introduction of a shorter double-curved catheter (only about nine inches long) through the wound into the bladder, where it should be left for three days. This seems to diminish the risk of rigors, and other symptoms of fever, which are apt to occur when the urine is allowed for the first time to pass over the wound.

Perineal Section is an operation both dangerous and difficult; as Sir Astley Cooper used to say, "the surgeon who performs it requires to have a long summer's day before him."

No director or guide can be passed. A full-sized catheter must be passed as far as possible up to the stricture, and held firmly in the middle line. The patient must be tied up in lithotomy position on a table in the very best light that can be obtained. The perineum being shaved, an incision must be made in the middle line from over the point of the catheter to the verge of the anus, if the stricture extends far back.

The urethra should then be opened over the catheter, the edges of the mucous membrane held to each side by silk threads passed through them; and the surgeon must endeavour to pass a fine probe into the opening of the stricture; if this can be done, it is comparatively easy to slit the stricture up. If not, the surgeon must simply seek for the remains of the urethra by slow, cautious dissection in the middle line. If successful, a catheter must be secured in the bladder in the usual way.

A stricture near the orifice, or, as it is not uncommon, involving merely the meatus, can be treated with great ease in the above manner by division on a grooved probe. When quite close to the orifice, with a well-defined hardness, as of a ring round the urethra, it may be divided subcutaneously by a tenotomy knife or other narrow-bladed

196

instrument. It is not necessary to keep a catheter in the bladder in cases where the stricture has been in front of the scrotum.

PUNCTURE OF THE BLADDER.—A patient and dexterous use of the catheter prevents this operation from being often required; still, circumstances may arise in which it is found impossible to enter the bladder per vias naturales. In such a case the bladder may be punctured from the outside by a curved trocar and canula, in either of two situations.

1. *From above the pubis.*—This operation is a very simple one, and when the bladder is distended need not imply a wound of the peritoneum.

Operation.—A preliminary incision, varying in length according to the amount of fat, should be made above the pubis exactly in the middle line; the edges of the recti should be separated, the peritoneum pushed out of the way and upwards by the finger, and a curved trocar plunged into the distended bladder obliquely backwards. The canula should be retained for a day or two, and then a flexible catheter with a shield inserted instead. Such instruments have been worn for years. The aspirateur pneumatique of Dr. Dieulafoy will be found an exceedingly useful instrument for puncture of bladder and removal of urine. The author has now used it very frequently with the best results. Its advantage is that the urine is removed through an aperture so small as to allow of the withdrawal and reintroduction of the canula as often as is necessary.

Fig. xxxvi.[157]

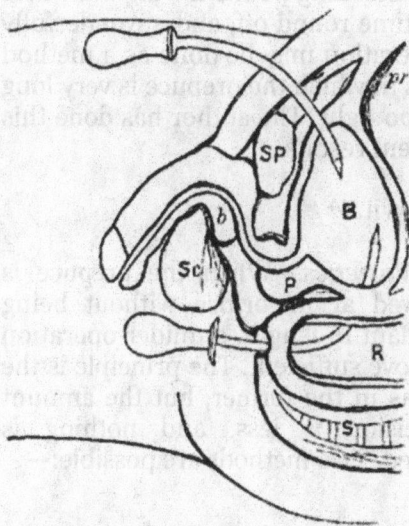

2. *From the Rectum.*— Except in cases of enlargement of the prostate, it is at once easier and safer to puncture the bladder from the rectum. The well-known triangular space uncovered by peritoneum, with its apex in front close to the prostate, and bounded on either side by the vasa deferentia and vesiculæ seminales, can be easily reached by a curved trocar. This should be guided by one, or, still better, by two fingers, into the rectum, with its concavity upwards, and the point should be pushed upwards by depression of the handle, whenever point should be pushed upwards by depression of the handle, whenever

---

[157] Diagram of puncture of the bladder:—b, bladder; sp, symphysis pubis; sc, scrotum; b, bulb; pr, peritoneum; p, prostate; r, rectum; s, sacrum and coccyx.

it is fairly behind the prostate. The trocar may then be withdrawn, and the canula retained for at least forty-eight hours by a suitable bandage. Mr. Cock, of Guy's Hospital, had a special canula for the purpose, which expands at its extremity after its introduction, and thus is not apt to slip.[158] Some surgeons insist that the surgeon should be able to ascertain the existence of fluctuation between the finger in the rectum, and the other hand above the pubes. This is exceedingly difficult to elicit when the bladder is very much distended, and from the constrained position of the finger in the bowel.

PHYMOSIS.—Elongation of the prepuce, with contraction of its orifice, in most cases congenital, sometimes so extreme as to cause difficulty in micturition, and frequently preventing the uncovering of the glans.

Operation.—In all well-marked cases, the following is required:— The elongated prepuce should be pulled forwards by a pair of catch-forceps, and a circle of skin and mucous membrane removed by a single stroke of a bistoury, or by sharp scissors. Care should be taken lest the glans be included in the incision, as has happened in at least one instance. The skin will then be found to retract very freely beyond the glans, but the mucous membrane is found still to cover the glans, and its orifice is still constricted. It must then be slit up (Fig. xxxvii. b b) on the dorsum of the glans, with probe-pointed scissors, as far as the corona, and the glans will then be thoroughly exposed. The edges of mucous membrane and skin should then be stitched to each other by at least five or six fine silk sutures, any bleeding points having been first carefully secured. The angles will in time round off, and a wonderfully seemly prepuce be obtained. This operation may be done as a method of cure for obstinate enuresis in cases in which the prepuce is very long and redundant, even when it is not too tight. The author has done this in more than twenty cases with excellent results.

Fig. xxxvii.[159]

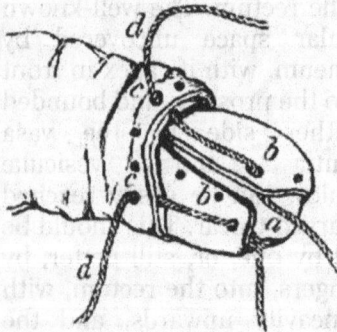

Varieties.—When the prepuce is narrowed at its orifice without being redundant in length, a milder operation will prove sufficient. The principle is the same as in the former, but the amount of incision is less, and nothing is removed. Two methods are possible:—

[158] Med. Chir. Trans., vol. xxxv.

[159] Diagram of operation for phymosis:—a, glans penis; b b, mucous membrane exposed by retraction of the skin, and slit up; c d, sutures introduced and ready to be tied, uniting the skin and mucous membrane.

1. *By scissors.*—The blunt point of a pair of scissors is introduced through the preputial orifice, the other blade being outside, and the skin and mucous membrane are divided for about half an inch; the skin being then retracted, the mucous membrane is still further divided by one or two additional snips, and then the edges of skin and mucous membrane are stitched together by one or two points of suture.

2. *By knife.*—A director being introduced within the prepuce, a narrow-bladed knife is guided along it, and pushed through the prepuce from within, and then made to divide skin and mucous membrane from within outwards. Stitches as before.

N.B.—Be careful lest the director pass into the meatus urinarius, and the glans be split up.

Again, some surgeons prefer two lateral incisions instead of one dorsal one. In this case skin and mucous membrane should be divided by scissors for about a quarter of an inch, and then a single stitch inserted in the angle of junction. This has been further modified by Cullerier, who proposed the division of the tight mucous membrane only, in three or four points. He used a pair of scissors with one sharp and one probe-pointed blade, the sharp one thrust in between skin and mucous membrane, the blunt one between the mucous membrane and the glans.

AMPUTATION OF THE PENIS.—This exceedingly simple operation is performed by a single stroke of an amputating knife, drawn along from heel to point, while the penis is stretched in the operator's left hand. As there is more risk of redundancy than of deficiency of the skin, no attempt is made to save it. Numerous vessels in the corpora cavernosa require ligature. Amputation of the penis may be done bloodlessly by the thermo-cautery even close to its root. Transfix the root of corpora cavernosa by a needle; above this pass two or three turns of an elastic ligature; then slowly divide at a low red heat the skin and corpora cavernosa below the needles; split the urethra after dividing its mucous membrane with a knife. The author has done this several times with ease and rapid healing.

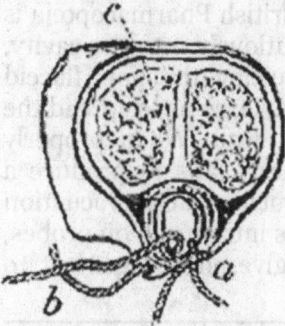

Fig. xxxviii.[160]

The chief risk is stricture of the orifice of the urethra. To prevent this, several modifications of the operation have been introduced.

1. *Ricord's method.*[161]—After the amputation the surgeon seizes with forceps

---

[160] To illustrate Teale's operation:—c, section of penis b, thread inserted uniting mucous membrane and skin; a, thread tied.

the mucous membrane of the urethra, and with a pair of scissors makes four slits in it, so as to form four equal flaps, and with a silk ligature stitches each of these to the skin. Contraction of the cicatrix will thus tend to open rather than close the urethral orifice.

2. *Teale's method.*[162]—He slits up, by a bistoury on a director, the urethra and skin over it for about two-thirds of an inch, and then stitches the one to the other, thus making it a long oval dependent orifice (Fig. xxxviii.).

3. *Miller's proposed method.*[163]—"A narrow-bladed knife is first used to transfix the penis between the spongy and cavernous bodies close to the root; the knife having been carried forwards for an inch and a half, its edge is turned perpendicularly downwards, and the urethra and skin flap are divided, the cavernous bodies and dorsal integument being then cut perpendicularly upwards where the knife was originally entered for transfixion. A button-hole is afterwards made in the lower flap, though which the corpus spongiosum and urethra protrude, while the flap itself is turned upwards, and attached dorsally and laterally, so as to cover in the exposed cavernous structure."

HYDROCELE.—The very simple operation necessary for hydrocele is thus performed:—The surgeon supports the tumour in his left hand so as to project it forwards, and make the scrotum as tense as possible in front. Having carefully ascertained the exact position of the testicle, which can generally be easily enough done by a finger accustomed to discriminate the difference between a soft solid, and a bag tensely filled with fluid, aided by the peculiar sensation of the testicle when squeezed, the surgeon enters a trocar and canula about an eighth of an inch in diameter into the distended cavity of the tunica vaginalis, near the fundus of the swelling. When it is evident the instrument is fairly entered, and not till then, the trocar is withdrawn, and the fluid allowed completely to drain off. When it ceases to flow the surgeon places his forefinger over the end of the canula to prevent the entrance of air, till he fits into its orifice a suitable syringe containing two drachms of the tincture of iodine, made according to the Edinburgh Pharmacopœia: the tincture of the British Pharmacopœia is not sufficiently strong. Having injected this cautiously into the cavity, the canula is withdrawn, and the surgeon, seizing the now flaccid scrotum in his right hand, gives it a thorough shake, so as to spread the iodine over as much as possible of the inner wall. When properly performed this very simple procedure very rarely fails to produce a radical cure; though less thorough operations, such as mere evacuation of the fluid, less stimulating injections, unguents introduced on probes, and the like, often fail of success, and thus give encouragement to

---

[161] Med. Times and Gazette, vol. xix. p. 354.
[162] Miller's System of Surgery, p. 1255.
[163] Miller's System of Surgery, p. 1256.

absurdities, such as wire-setons, or to more severe operations, such as laying open the sac.

HÆMATOCELE.—When the contents of the sac of the tunica vaginalis are found to be grumous instead of simply serous, or when, as often happens, only pure blood escapes when the fluid is nearly evacuated, it is found that simple evacuation and injection are very rarely sufficient to effect a cure.

After they have been fairly tried, the sac of the hæmatocele should be laid open in its full extent; any large vessels which bleed should be tied, and the cavity then stuffed with lint. When the lint can be removed, which will be after two or three days, the edges of the wound should be brought closely together, and the cavity will then rapidly heal up from the bottom, and be obliterated by secondary union of granulations.

In cases where the walls of the cavity are enormously thickened, or even, as sometimes happens, almost bony in consistence, an elliptical portion may be removed with advantage.

EXCISION OF TESTICLE.—This operation is rarely required except for tumours of the testicle. Hence the size of the incision necessary must vary much with the size of the tumour; and the amount of skin to be removed (if any) on the amount of adhesions it has formed to the tumour.

One or two points must be attended to in every case of extirpation of a testicle:—

1. The incision should commence over the cord just outside of the external ring, and be continued fairly over the tumour to its base.

2. As to removal of skin, some surgeons advise that none should be taken away, others that a considerable quantity can be spared. There is certainly less risk of secondary hæmorrhage if a portion be removed, than when a flaccid empty bag is left. The author invariably removes a very large quantity of skin if the tumour is large, as there is much more rapid healing, and the resulting scrotum is much more comfortable for the patient.

3. The cord should be exposed at the beginning of the operation, raised from its bed and given to an assistant, who should compress it gently, not from any fear of its escape into the abdomen, but to prevent hæmorrhage. If the tumour has been very large and heavy, the cord will have been much stretched, and if divided too high up, may really give trouble by its elasticity, unless the above precaution is taken. The cord then having been divided close to the tumour, the latter is removed, care being taken not to include the sound testicle in the removal. All the vessels are then to be tied or twisted, and the spermatic artery is to be secured alone, not, as used to be the case, included in a common ligature with the other constituents of the cord. Secondary hæmorrhage is very apt to occur from small scrotal branches which may have escaped notice during the operation.

OPERATIONS ON THE ANUS AND ITS NEIGHBOURHOOD.—

FISTULA IN ANO.—While much might be written on the pathology of fistula, and a good deal even on its diagnosis, a very few words will suffice to describe the simple and effectual operation for its relief.

Dismissing at once all so-called palliatives, drugs, unguents, pressure, and injections, as mere waste of time, and holding that the only method of cure consists in laying the fistula fairly open, the question narrows itself into this: What is the best method of laying it open? Prior to the discovery by Ribes of the great principle that the internal orifice of the sinus is always within an inch or an inch and a half of the orifice of the anus, the operations for fistula were most unnecessarily severe; the gut used to be divided as far up as the sinuses extended; and large portions of the anus used to be excised bodily along with the sinuses. It is now a much simpler and more satisfactory operation.

Operation.—A common silver probe bent to the required shape is passed into the external opening, or, if there are more than one, into the largest and oldest one. The forefinger of the left hand being introduced into the rectum, the probe is passed through the internal orifice, and its point brought out by the anus. The portion of tissue raised by the probe can then be easily divided with the certainty that the fistula is laid fully open. Anal fistulæ have been divided by the elastic ligature, but it seems slower in action and more painful, with no counterbalancing advantages.

The author has for last few years operated almost exclusively by a long knife which is continued into a steel probe. The probe is passed up the fistula, then into the bowel, and is hooked out at the anus, and in being simply pushed on the knife cuts the fistula—tuto, cito, et jucunde, the patient rarely knowing that more has been done than an exploration.

In cases where, from the hardness and density of the parts it is impossible to pass the probe and bring it out at the anus, a strong probe-pointed bistoury may be passed in by the external orifice till its probe-point can be felt by the finger in the bowel at the internal opening. Supported by the finger it can then be made to cut outwards till the whole septum is divided.

FISSURE OF THE ANUS, ULCER OF THE ANUS, resemble each other alike in the exceeding annoyance which they give to the sufferer, and in the simplicity of the treatment needed.

Operation.—Once the presence of either is determined by the finger in the anus, a sharp-pointed curved bistoury should be introduced, transfixing the base of the fissure or ulcer, and then guided on the finger, completely dividing it, so as to change the ragged ulceration into a simple wound which will rapidly heal.

PROLAPSUS ANI, *Operation for.*—Complete prolapsus in which the whole gut is involved, as seen in the very young and the very aged, is suited for palliative rather than radical treatment.

Cases of prolapsus of the mucous membrane only, as is not uncommon in connection with or as a result of hæmorrhoids in adults, give opportunity for operative interference.

We may act on either the skin or mucous membrane, or both at once.

1. *The skin* is often found loose, and arranged in radiating folds round the anus. In such cases, as recommended first by Dupuytren, some of these projecting folds may be removed. Again it may be prolapsed in a great loose ring or circular fold round the margin, forming an exaggerated external pile; in such a case the loose fold may be fairly excised with curved scissors, as recommended by Hey of Leeds.

The first of these methods is apt to be insufficient, the second again has the risk of removing too much.

2. If the protrusion is chiefly mucous membrane exposed in folds, or a ring, which is generally outside, one of two methods of treatment may be tried:—

a. By ligature, as recommended by Mr. Copeland. Raising a longitudinal fold of the mucous membrane, he passed a ligature round it as if it were a pile. There is less chance of the ligature slipping if a double thread be used and its base thus transfixed. Three, four, or even more folds may be thus treated.

b. When the mucous membrane has been so long exposed as to have lost many of its characters, and to resemble leather in its toughness, excision will be found less painful and much more rapid than ligature.

A longitudinal fold at each side of the anus should be pinched up and excised by a pair of probe-pointed curved scissors. There is always a certain amount of risk of hæmorrhage following such an operation. The risk is lessened and the result improved by stitching up the wound in the mucous membrane before the protruded portion of bowel is returned.

POLYPI OF THE RECTUM.—Pedunculated growths varying in consistence, shape, and size, but resembling each other in having a distinct stalk, and in frequently being protruded at stool.

Operation.—Invariably by ligature, which may be single round the stalk, if the tumour be globular and with a distinct narrow stalk, or by transfixion, if (as sometimes happens) the tumour be of uniform thickness throughout, like a worm.

HÆMORRHOIDS OR PILES.—In the treatment of piles it is the differential diagnosis that is troublesome and occasionally difficult; the operative interference required is generally very simple, if the nature of the case be rightly determined.

External piles.—Operation.—The apex of the soft flabby excrescence should be seized by a pair of catch-forceps, and it should be cut off close to its base with a knife, or, what is better, a pair of curved scissors. Any little vessel which jets may then be secured. If,

203

instead of numerous individual tumours, a ring of skin round the anus be involved, the whole of it should be shaved off, but not very close to its base, lest too great contraction of the anal orifice should ensue.

If the surgeon, after excising a pile or piles, will take the trouble to stitch up the wound with catgut, he will find the cure much more rapid and less painful than when this is omitted.

Internal piles.—Incision is extremely dangerous, from the vascularity of the parts, and their being so inaccessible from their position within the sphincter ani. Hence ligature is safer and equally effectual. The patient should be directed to sit over hot water, and strain till the whole of his piles are fairly protruded. The surgeon should then transfix the base of each separately with a curved needle bearing a strong double thread. The needle being cut off, the threads should be very firmly tied, each isolating its own half of the pile. The tying should be exceedingly tight, so as to cause instant and complete strangulation and death of the tumours. All the piles should be tied at the same sitting. If the piles are very small they may be secured without transfixion in a single noose after being seized by a hook or forceps. There is greater risk of the noose slipping than when the base has been transfixed.

The strangulated masses must then be returned into the bowel, and the patient kept in bed or on a sofa till the ligatures separate, which is generally not till the fourth or fifth day. A certain amount of urinary irritation, showing itself sometimes in strangury, sometimes in complete retention, occasionally follows this operation.

Mr. Smith of King's College, and many other surgeons, treat internal piles by means of an ivory clamp to hold them tight, while they are burned off by the actual cautery or the thermo-cautery at a low red heat. They claim that pyæmia more rarely follows this mode.

There are certain cases in which the lower inch or two of the rectum are found red and congested, and in which every stool is followed by the loss of a certain quantity of florid arterial blood, and yet no distinct hæmorrhoidal tumour is to be seen. In such cases the ligature is not applicable, and relief is obtained by the application of pure nitric acid, or other potential caustics to the bleeding surface, as recommended by Houston, Lee, Smith, Ashton, and others. These cases are comparatively rare, and whenever they can be applied, the ligature is much simpler, safer, and more certain.

Venous piles.—When a sudden effusion of blood has occurred into one of the varicose veins or sinuses of a congested anus, an oval or rounded tumour is felt, very tense, shining, and painful. To slit it freely up with an abscess lancet, and evert the clot inside, at once relieves all the symptoms.

204

CHAPTER XIII

TENOTOMY

For convenience' sake I group under this one head certain operations used for the relief of distortion, in which muscles or tendons are divided subcutaneously. Since the discovery of the principle by Delpech, and the application of it by Stromeyer, Dieffenbach, Little, and countless successors, it has been used for very many cases for which it is totally inapplicable, e.g. for the division of the muscles of the back in spinal curvature. Still there remain several deformities for the relief of which subcutaneous tenotomy is a most important remedy; chief among these are Wry Neck and Club-foot.

OPERATION FOR WRY NECK.—Subcutaneous section of the sterno-mastoid.—In what cases of wry neck is this operation suitable? In those only in which the muscles are the starting-point of the mischief. These are sometimes congenital, more frequently they commence in childhood. In cases where the distortion depends on disease of the cervical vertebræ, or is secondary to curvature of the spine, division of the muscle is worse than useless.

Operation.—A tenotomy knife, which should be sharp-pointed, narrow in the blade, with a blunt back, should be introduced through the skin a little to one side of the sternal portion of the affected muscle, passed along with its flat edge between the skin and the tendon, till it has fairly crossed the tendon; the blade should then be turned so that by a gradual sawing motion the edge may be made to divide the tendon about an inch above the sternum. A distinct snap will then be felt or heard, and the position of the head will be at once much improved. Exercise, warm bathing, and rubbing, will generally suffice to complete the cure, without it being necessary to call in the aid of the instrument-maker with his expensive apparatus.[164]

OPERATIONS FOR CLUB-FOOT.—The following are the tendons which may require division in the cure of club-foot, and the operations for their division.

1. The tendo Achillis.—There are very few cases of true club-foot which can be successfully treated without division of the tendo Achillis. While in talipes equinis it is generally the only disturbing agent, in talipes varus and valgus it invariably increases and maintains the deformity, which the tibiales or peronei seem to originate.

Operation.—The foot being held at about a right angle with the leg, the operator should pinch up the skin over the tendon, introduce

---

[164] Syme's Pathology and Practice of Surgery, p. 220.

the knife flatwise, a little to one side of the tendon, till its point is nearly projecting at the other, then turn the edge on the tendon and cut inwards with a sawing motion till the tendon gives way with a distinct snap, and the foot can be completely flexed with ease.

Dr. Little[165] recommends that the tendon should be divided from before backwards. There is more risk by this method of wounding the skin, and thus losing the subcutaneous character of the operation.

Professor Pancoast[166] divides the inferior portion of the soleus muscle instead of the tendo Achillis.

2. *Tibialis posticus.*—Next in frequency and importance to that of the tendo Achillis, division of this tendon is much more difficult to perform. It may be performed either above or below the ankle.

(a.) *Above the ankle.*—The blade of a tenotomy knife should be entered perpendicularly at the posterior margin of the tibia, half an inch or an inch above the internal malleolus, so as to pass between the bone and the tendon of the tibialis posticus, the blade directed towards the latter; the assistant should now evert the foot, the operator pressing the blade against the tendon.[167]

(b.) *Below the ankle, close to the attachment to the scaphoid.* This is the better position of the two when the position of the tendon can be made out, which is not always the case, especially in cases of old standing.

Raising the skin just over the astragalo-scaphoid joint, the knife should be entered with its blade downwards, and across the tendon, and should be made to cut on the bone, while an assistant everts the foot till the tendon gives way with a distinct snap.

3. *Tibialis anticus* may in like manner be divided either just above the ankle, or at its insertion. When it requires division it can generally be made so prominent as to render its division comparatively easy.

4. *Peronei.*—These do not often require division, cases of talipes valgus being usually paralytic in character. If necessary they can be cut as they cross the fibula.

5. *The plantar fascia*, may require division; when this is the case, it is so prominent as to render the operation very easy, if conducted on the principles mentioned above.

---

[165] Holmes's Surgery, vol. iii. p. 573.
[166] Cross's Surgery, vol. ii. p. 273, 3d ed.
[167] Miller's System of Surgery, p. 1339; Holmes's Surgery, vol. iii. p. 571.

CHAPTER XIV

OPERATIONS ON NERVES

NERVE-STRETCHING.—Surgical literature in last ten years is full of cases in which nerves have been stretched for all manner of diseases with varying success: an example of the operative procedure may suffice:—

1. Stretching of the great sciatic either for sciatica, sclerosis, or locomotor ataxia.

Operation.—A line drawn from the centre of the space between the tuberosity of the ischium or the great trochanter to a corresponding point between the condyles of the femur will give the direction. A free incision in this line three or four inches in length—the nerve lies just below the the femoral aponeurosis, beneath the edge of gluteal fold, requiring no muscular fibres to be divided. It must be raised from its bed and boldly stretched or elongated into a loop. Symington's experiments have shown that in the average adult 130 lb. are required to break the nerve.

2. The facial has been stretched for spasm. The trunk is easily reached by an incision extending from near the external auditory meatus to the angle of the jaw, which enables the parotid to be pushed forward and the edge of the sterno-mastoid pulled backwards.

NEUROTOMY AND NEURECTOMY.—Chiefly performed for neuralgia of the fifth nerve.

a. This is a very easy operation if directed at the terminal branches only of the nerve, where they make their exit from the frontal, supraorbital, and mental foramina. The author has done it in very numerous cases, and with great relief, if care be taken to destroy the nerve in the foramen to some extent—a sharp-pointed thermo-cautery does this easily and safely.

b. The more severe and radical operation of cutting out a portion of the trunk of the fifth nerve just after it has left the skull, and destroying Meckel's ganglion, has been done pretty frequently, chiefly by American surgeons—in various ways.

1. *Carnochan's Operation.*—Exposing the whole front wall of antrum, its cavity is opened into from the front by a large trephine. The lower wall of the infra-orbital canal is cut away by a chisel, the posterior wall of the antrum by a smaller trephine, the nerve thus isolated is traced up to and past Meckel's ganglion, which is removed close to the foramen rotundum by cutting the nerve by curved blunt-pointed scissors.

2. *Pancoast's Operation.*—Expose the coronoid process by a free

207

incision, divide it at its root and throw it up, then expose and tie internal maxillary artery, after which the upper portion of the external pterygoid is to be detached from the sphenoid, thus exposing the nerve leaving foramen ovale; the second portion is deeper and not so easily got at.

3. The spinal accessory occasionally may be divided before it enters the sterno-mastoid in cases of spasmodic wry neck, with great advantage. This operation is an easy one; the sterno-mastoid edge being once fairly exposed, the nerve is easily seen, and a piece should be cut out at least half an inch in length.

Nerve Suture is occasionally practised with great advantage in cases where nerves have been divided either by accident or in operation. Catgut seems to be the best medium, and cases are on record in which, even after months of separation and subsequent paralysis, improvement has followed an operation for refreshing and joining the divided ends.

ADDENDUM TO CHAPTER IX

Dr. Solis Cohen has recently (in a paper read before the Philadelphia College of Physicians, April 4, 1883) collected the notes of sixty-five cases of excision of the entire larynx. Fifty-six of these were done for cancer, and the remainder for sarcomata, papillomata, etc. Of the fifty-six done for cancer, forty are reported as having died, either shortly after the operation from shock or pneumonia, or a few months later from recurrence of the disease. In two instances the disease had recurred, but death had not been reported when the paper was read. Fourteen remain in which neither death nor recurrence had been reported. Dr. Cohen's conclusion is that laryngectomy does not tend to the prolongation of life, and thinks that the greatest good to the greater number appears better secured by dependence on the palliative operation of tracheotomy.